Porn Panic!

Sex and Censorship in the UK

Porn Panic!

Sex and Censorship in the UK

Jerry Barnett

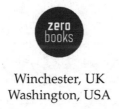

Winchester, UK
Washington, USA

First published by Zero Books, 2016
Zero Books is an imprint of John Hunt Publishing Ltd., Laurel House, Station Approach,
Alresford, Hants, SO24 9JH, UK
office1@jhpbooks.net
www.johnhuntpublishing.com
www.zero-books.net

For distributor details and how to order please visit the 'Ordering' section on our website.

Text copyright: Jerry Barnett 2015

ISBN: 978 1 78535 374 1
Library of Congress Control Number: 2015960668

A CIP catalogue record for this book is available from the British Library.

Design: Lee Nash

Printed and bound by CPI Group (UK) Ltd, Croydon, CR0 4YY, UK

CONTENTS

1

Introduction

censor [sen-ser] (noun): any person who supervises the manners or morality of others

Given the family and environment I was born into, it was virtually inevitable I would become immersed in political activism. My grandfather Albert Mann (later Albert Mann MBE), as a young Jewish man growing up in London's East End ghettos, had been politicised by the rise of fascism, as well as by the poverty that surrounded him during his childhood. When the fascist leader Oswald Mosley tried to lead his blackshirts through the Jewish East End on 4th October 1936, Albert was one of many thousands who came out onto the streets to block Mosley's progress. Jews, other locals and communists united to physically beat the blackshirts out of the East End. Women threw heavy pots out of windows onto fascist heads. The police deployed their truncheons against the protesters, but were beaten back, along with the fascists. This victory of the left, known as the Battle of Cable Street, was a turning point in the fight against British fascism.

The mainstream parties of left and right failed to either fully understand or strongly oppose fascism, and so in the 1930s many progressives (including Albert) joined the only strongly anti-fascist force, the Communist Party, which became a mass political party for the next two decades. During WWII, Albert fought in the RAF against fascism, and was among the returning soldiers who voted for the most left-wing government in British history. The Labour victory of 1945 secured the foundation of the National Health Service, the welfare state and universal education, institutions which Albert fought to defend for the remainder of his life (although, like many former communists, he was eventually repelled by Stalinism and found his lifelong home in the Labour Party).

Albert's stridently progressive views politicised his daughter, my mother. She was of the 1960s generation of young people attracted by second-wave feminism (known at the time as the Women's Lib movement), which campaigned for equal rights for women, and in particular for sexual liberation. Some of the first sexual writing I encountered, in my prepubescent years, was in the pages of my mum's feminist magazines, such as *Spare Rib*. In such publications, women were told that they had a right to sexual pleasure, and were advised on how they might achieve it; men were teased for not being able to locate clitorises.

Post-Women's Lib, many women were no longer ashamed to reveal their bodies, and sexual imagery became more daring and less censored. In more liberated countries than Britain – led by Denmark in 1969 – pornography was decriminalised. Social and religious conservatives watched in horror as carefully constructed walls of censorship and anti-sex morality were swept away.

In her father's footsteps, my mum was also involved with the anti-fascist movement. In the 1970s, support for the National Front was surging, driven by concern about mass immigration. My mum took me to marches with her; the first I remember was a counter-protest against a march by an obscure far-right group, the British Movement, which had gained some popularity in West London. Perhaps a few hundred fascists had turned up, but there were tens of thousands of us, of all races, standing against them, and we prevented them from marching. On a smaller, gentler scale, I was repeating my grandfather's experience in Cable Street, four decades earlier.

In the late-1970s, the Rock Against Racism movement was combining the music of my generation – reggae, punk, ska – with anti-fascist politics, and mobilising a new generation into politics. We went to music festivals and on political marches. Rastafarians danced to the same music as skinheads, and racial divisions began to break down. The transformation of Britain's race relations was remarkably fast: the 1990s was a palpably different era from the 70s.

My political upbringing and my own activism meant that I spent my teens surrounded by activists from around the world: leading ANC exiles, fighting Apartheid from their temporary base in London; the children of left-wing activists who had fled state terror in Chile; political refugees from Zimbabwe, Mexico and dozens of other places. It was a dangerous, unsettled period, but an exciting time to be young, and in London. The alternative comedy scene was born, in small comedy clubs and rooms above pubs, giving us a welcome antidote to the stuffy, state-approved comedy on TV. The new comedy was left-wing, sweary, anti-establishment and sexually explicit. I joined one of the many Trotskyist organisations, the Militant Tendency. Riots erupted in inner cities; first in 1979, then more widespread in 1981. The early-80s felt like a revolutionary era, and we believed we were the vanguard of a socialist revolution that was about to sweep the globe.

But we were not, and it did not. Margaret Thatcher's historic defeat of the miners' strike in 1985 marked the end of the power of the proletariat, which was supposed to overthrow global capitalism. The industrial working class was vanishing. Many of the left-wing activists of my generation drifted away from politics. By then I had a young son, a family to support, and the beginnings of a career as a software developer. I felt, a little guiltily, that I was abandoning the revolution. As it turned out, I was joining it.

In 1988, working as a software engineer and technical consultant, I was allocated my first Internet email address. Here was a novelty: I could send text anywhere in the world, to anyone else on the Internet, and it would reach them quickly, often within minutes or even seconds! Most of the people I knew on the Net worked in the same building as me, but still, this was a revolutionary concept. I knew a couple of people in the United States with email addresses. Previously, we might have spoken or written to each other once a year, if that; now we could exchange messages on a daily basis. What is now normal was then a leap forward in global communication with mind-blowing implications.

The Internet continued to spread. Technology graduates left university wanting to stay in touch with their old email buddies. In the early-90s, some of these geeks set up the first companies to offer cheap dial-up access for home users. I joined one of these providers – Demon Internet – which offered a service for £10 per month. The Internet was still exclusively a place for techies; but then Tim Berners-Lee, a British scientist, launched a suite of software he had developed for easily publishing and sharing documents, which he called the World Wide Web. Now, people with minimal technical skills could publish information, and anyone could access it. In the slang of the day, we were all joining the Information Superhighway, or alternatively had become members of the Global Village.

The network had the potential to change everything, but perhaps its first significant effect was to reveal the true inner workings of the human mind. Now that anybody, with minimal money or skill, could publish whatever they liked, the Internet became a readable map of human thoughts. And, it turned out that, far more than anything else, we were interested in sex.

This fact should not have surprised anyone, but few people would have predicted the sheer scale of this new sexual revolution. In the first few years of the web, most of the Internet's capacity was dedicated to sexual hookups, erotic stories, sexual chat and information, and most of all, to pornography.

In 1994, I set up a web software business. Finally, computing was cool rather than nerdy, and I wanted to be involved with the new technologies. I quickly acquired customers, and recruited staff. One of my early clients was a pornographer who wanted to try selling explicit porn photos online; I built the site for him, it went live, and within a couple of years was one of the most trafficked sites on the web, for a time even outranking the BBC. Having entered the market so early, my client made a lot of money in a short space of time. Inevitably, others noticed, and a gold rush started. Hundreds of thousands, then millions of porn sites appeared online in the late-90s and early-noughties. As the dot-com crash of 2000 came and went, many of the weird and wonderful startups of the early web vanished; this served to highlight the fact that, at that time, there was only one big, profitable online industry. As many fledgling web businesses lost their investors and closed down, porn continued to grow from strength to strength.

All of this took place during a liberal upswing in British culture. The 90s was a decade when Britain turned its back on the gloomy, authoritarian Thatcher era; dance music and ecstasy-fuelled ravers took over from power ballads and cocaine-fuelled yuppies. The Cold War, with its nuclear nightmares, faded away. Sex became freer, sexuality more liberated, racial mixing more common. A Labour government was elected after 18 years of Tory rule, and quickly updated laws to match the new zeitgeist. Anti-gay legislation was repealed, civil partnerships were intro- duced, and the age of consent for homosexuals was reduced from 21 to 18, and then 16. Cash-starved public services were properly funded again. Newly built schools and hospitals appeared. The homeless evaporated from the streets of London. The economy was growing after years of recession and stagnation, and people had more money in their pockets.

In the background, conservative forces were biding their time. Since the 1970s, the British state had been carefully assembling a raft of censorship laws, regulations and bodies to ensure that the British public could only see and hear officially approved material. No other democratic country had such tight controls over the media. Most of all, the state abhorred sexual expression: *No Sex Please, We're British* definitely applied to our media regulators, if not to the average Brit anymore. In particular, they had ensured that hard-core pornography was virtually inaccessible. It had been completely banned from television (indeed, it still is), and also from video and DVD. Via unlicensed sex shops, car-boot sales and blokes in pubs, one could buy pirate porn videos, but they were illegal to supply, and expensive (a friend involved in the business at the time reminisces about selling pirated VHS tapes for £70).

The walls of British censorship began to be breached with the launch of satellite TV: hard-core porn was broadcast from Denmark, and British subscribers signed up in droves. The government quickly moved to ban the sale of the required receivers. Low-cost airlines began trading, and suddenly Brits could pop over to Amsterdam, Hamburg or Barcelona for the weekend. Many returned carrying porn videos far more explicit than those legally available in the UK.

And the web began to seriously erode the powers of the British censorship state. Censorship laws, such as the ancient Obscene Publications Act, were aimed at suppliers, not consumers. But now the suppliers were overseas, beyond the short reach of British jurisdiction. The highly censorious TV regulators (which were eventually merged into one super-regulator, Ofcom) had no jurisdiction over the Internet; neither did the BBFC, which only had a remit to censor physical media such as video and DVD. With the new century came faster Internet connections, capable of delivering streaming video; the early adoption of broadband was, in large part, driven by porn consumers: there was almost no other content available to watch online at that stage. In a remarkably short period of time, the British censorship state largely lost its ability to control which media could be consumed by British citizens. The United States and most of the European Union had far laxer laws regarding pornography than the UK, and for the first time in our history, the British people could not be deprived of explicit sexual expression. No wonder we binged.

In 2004, after building porn sites for other businesses for almost a decade, I launched my own video service, Strictly Broadband, which sold rentals of porn DVDs in online streaming form (it was somewhat similar in approach to later services like Netflix). As I became more involved with the adult entertainment industry, I became increasingly aware of two trends: first, there was a new morality movement on the rise; the liberalism of the 90s generation was fading. And second, the British state was well aware of the rising threat to its power, and was preparing to claw it back, using pornography as one of the key excuses for taking draconian action (terrorism being another favoured excuse, in the wake of 9/11). Both of these trends – the new moralists, and state censorship – began to worry me, and to draw me back again towards political involvement. In 2008, the financial crash led to an upsurge in activism, as a new left-wing generation – the first since the 1980s – became involved in battling a Conservative-led government.

The old anti-sex movement, led by the vociferous, veteran decency campaigner Mary Whitehouse, had become a laughing stock, a memory of more religious and uptight generations. When Whitehouse died, in 2001, it had seemed to herald the end of an era. What I missed at the time, and discovered later, was that Whitehouse's death had left a space for the arrival of a new morality movement. The old moralists had wielded the Bible in one hand, and the *Daily Mail* in the other. This new movement was younger. Instead of coming from Middle England, it arrived from academia. Rather than use the language of religious morality, it appeared under the umbrella of feminism and liberalism. And in place of the *Mail*, it was backed by the *Guardian*. Just like Whitehouse, these new activists hated pornography most of all, and blamed it for many of the world's (often imaginary) ills.

For me, emerging blinking back into the world of political activism after a couple of decades, this was disorientating. I was a Labour-voting (well, until Iraq anyway), *Guardian*-reading leftie; what had happened to my tribe? I had believed that the new, secular Britain had left behind the old conservative attitudes about sex and sexuality; but instead, the anti-sex tendency had merely lain dormant, redefined itself for a new era, and waited for its time to come. I had thought the decline of organised religion would bring about the end of moralists who sought to control other people's private behaviours. I was wrong: the fear of sex, and the power to control populations using sexual repression, are far older and more primal instincts than mere religion or politics.

I sought to become involved in campaigning against censorship, and discovered that there is little that could be described as an anti-censorship movement in the UK. I found myself almost alone in a parliamentary inquiry, trying to convince MPs that censorship – whether of pornography or anything else – is antithetical to democracy and to liberal values. It was dispiriting indeed to discover how deeply a fear of free expression had become embedded in British culture and politics, not just on the right, but at least as much on the left.

Left and right are not tied to permanent sets of principles, but are mere labels; ever-changing statements of tribal identity. This is hardly a new observation: George Orwell, always ahead of his time, understood the fluidity of political identity better than anyone when he wrote in closing *Animal Farm*: "The creatures outside looked from pig to man, and from man to pig, and from pig to man again, but already it was impossible to say which was which". Orwell also noted the conservatism inherent within the left in *1984*: the ruling clique was known as Ingsoc – an abbreviation for the English Socialist Party. Young people were encouraged to join the Junior Anti-Sex League, "which advocated complete celibacy for both sexes... The Party was trying to kill the sex instinct, or if it could not be killed, then to distort it and dirty it".

This book, *Porn Panic!*, documents the neo-puritans, their origins, and the numerous moral panics they have sown in recent years. These panics have been supported by a wide variety of players, each with their own reasons for wanting to put free expression, and most of all sexual expression, back in its box. Ultimately their collective aim is to create the conditions for something that has not yet occurred in any democratic country: wide-scale, state-enforced censorship of the Internet. They do this by making the case that, when it comes to expression, there are some lines that simply must not be crossed, and that therefore the state must intervene in public discourse.

I will show that evidence that pornography causes harm simply does not exist; but I will also make the case that, even if porn had proved to be in some way harmful, censorship is far more harmful. Empowering the state to control our speech has been done many times, for many reasons, and rarely (if ever) with good outcomes. It is tempting to think we can merely censor the 'bad stuff' while allowing the 'good stuff' to get through: but this is not possible. To accept state censorship is to empower the state to decide which expression it will act against next. We should allow the state new powers with the greatest caution, or regret at leisure. In the words of the great Enlightenment thinker Benjamin Franklin: "Those who will give up essential Liberty, to purchase a little temporary Safety, deserve neither Liberty nor Safety".

2

40,000 Years of Porn

And the man and his wife were both naked and were not ashamed –
Genesis 2:25

*And the Lord God made for Adam and for his wife garments of skins
and clothed them –* Genesis 3:21

The first problem one encounters in writing about pornography is to define what it is; the term is often used as a derogatory one, as a label for any form of sexual expression that is considered too gratuitous, too crude or lacking in artistic or intellectual value by the viewer to be labelled art. Thus, almost any form of expression, artistic or otherwise, that is related to sexuality, is pornographic from some person's viewpoint. 'Pornography' is the insult that is thrown at the work that the viewer considers offensive; and since offence is in the eye of the beholder, any sexual work is potentially pornographic.

The late American pornstar and porn-maker Kelly Steele, who I knew when she lived in London, believed that in order to be pornographic, a work must be shocking, and so the duty of a true pornographer must be to continually test society's tolerance for what can be 'acceptable'. However, artists in many other fields also set themselves this objective: to shock and to test the bounds of societal morals and taboos could be said to be a function of all art, not just that narrow selection that, instinctively, we label as pornographic.

The UK's film censor, the British Board of Film Classification (BBFC) has two categories for content it deems to be potentially harmful to children: a work that is considered pornographic (but within the bounds of UK obscenity law) may be awarded an R18 certificate, meaning it can only be distributed via one of the UK's 400 or so licensed sex shops, or shown in a licensed adult cinema. It is illegal to sell an R18 (or unclassified) work via mail order. A softer title, featuring simulated or hidden sex acts, may receive an 18 certificate, meaning that it can be put out for general cinematic release, and sold via unlicensed shops and by mail order.

The boundary between 18 and R18, however, is a complex one; explicit sex acts may feature in films that, because the censor deems them to have some artistic merit, still receive an 18 certificate and are therefore approved for general cinematic release. The 2000 French film *Baise Moi*, featuring an explicit rape scene, and *9 Songs* (2004) including multiple hard-core sex scenes, were both awarded 18 certificates. A particular sexual act in one context may be approved for cinematic release, while an identical scene in a different context may only be available on DVD in sex shops. British people are generally unaware that the decision as to what is – or is not – artistic still lies in the hands of government-appointed censors, rather than with art commentators or the general public. Furthermore, we fund these acts of censorship, and they are carried out in the name of protecting us, the public. Britain is one of the most censored nations in the democratic world; and is becoming more so.

The definition of pornography therefore changes depending on who is viewing it, and when. As mass communication becomes more open, we fail to be shocked by things that might have been considered too much by previous generations.

None of this takes us much further in defining porn; it apparently refers to any sexual expression, some sexual expression, or nothing at all, depending on whose eyes we are looking through. The best definition, perhaps, was famously provided by the US Supreme Court Justice Potter Stewart in 1964 when he declared:

I shall not today attempt further to define the kinds of material I understand to be embraced within that shorthand description ["hard-core pornography"]; and perhaps I could never succeed in intelligibly doing so. But I know it when I see it...

In a world of free expression, this definition would work just fine, were it not for one small problem: some people (whatever their stated or actual objectives may be) feel the need to control and restrict the personal lives of others. While most people may be happy to enjoy pornography (or erotica, or sexual art), and to allow others to do so, it only takes a small, active minority to impose controls over the lives of the majority.

The histories of artistic expression, sexual expression, sexuality, free speech and political freedom are intimately entwined with each other; an attack on any of these freedoms is an attack on them all. Sexual expression is often declared to be the 'canary in the coal mine': while many attack porn because they genuinely dislike or fear it, for authoritarians, it is simply chosen because it is a soft and hard-to-defend target. Put into place a legal and regulatory regime that ostensibly exists to censor pornography, and controls on other expression can and will follow.

As for my definition of pornography: I use it to mean any form of expression that somebody could find sexually stimulating. I tend to use terms like 'porn', 'erotica' and 'sexual expression' interchangeably, since in practise they mean the same thing, especially to those who choose to attack our right to enjoy them.

When I refer to porn I am not including images and videos of nonconsensual acts such as rape and child abuse. Consenting adult sexual behaviour is not equivalent to, and should not be compared with, sexual violence; those who try to blur this obvious distinction should be treated with suspicion.

Ice-Age Pornography

Some of the earliest known human artworks were pornographic.

Many variants of carved Venus figurines or Mother Goddesses, some estimated to have been made up to 40,000 years ago, have been discovered across much of the Old World (in fact, disputed Venuses discovered in North Africa and the Middle East may date back as far as 500,000 years). These carvings typically display a curvaceous female form with a clear focus on feminine sexuality.

Art of the Ice Age, an exhibition at the British Museum which opened in February 2013, featured mankind's oldest known art – much of which is straightforwardly erotic. The exhibition included the oldest known ceramic work, the Venus of Dolní Věstonice, a piece made at least 25,000 years ago, and discovered in (what is now) the Czech Republic. This Venus features an obviously erotic female figure with exaggerated breasts and buttocks but with little attention paid to other, apparently less important, features like a face or arms.

The Wikipedia page on Mother Goddesses drily states: "Some archaeologists believe they were intended to represent goddesses, while others believe that they could have served some other purpose". It is not hard to guess what that "other purpose" might be; although sexually explicit figures like Mother Goddesses may evolve to be used in sacred rituals over time, it is difficult to deny that they, like all erotic art that followed, would have been of value because of their sexually stimulating nature; yet contemporary commentators, looking back at the pornography of ancient times, will tend to play on its 'sacred' and 'spiritual' nature, while taking care to avoid mention of its probable masturbatory purposes.

While all societies exhibit some degree of squeamishness in dealing with sexual expression in their present, commentators tend to explain away ancient sexual expression by ascribing noble intentions to the people who made it. At other times, ancient porn is simply censored, hidden away or destroyed completely. In these ways, puritans continually try to rewrite mankind's history – sanitised, with the sex removed. Perhaps future archaeologists, stumbling across the universal 'spunking cock' symbol with which today's schoolboys happily decorate toilet walls, will conduct earnest debates about the use of fertility symbols in our society; or discovering a stash of hard-core porn magazines, they will enthuse about our civilisation's 'spiritual' appreciation of the nubile female form. Regardless of the meanings we might ascribe to specific instances of sexual imagery, its regular reappearance across time and geography is undeniable; humans, for as long as we have had the technology to express anything artistically, have shown a particular interest in depicting sexuality.

The Venus figurines, first carved from stone and later sculpted from ceramics, are just the first of many examples of a phenomenon that repeats throughout history and prehistory: whenever communications technology has taken a leap forward, from ancient carving to the Internet, it invariably leads to a new explosion of sexual expression, a new sexual revolution. The appearance of writing for the first time, over 5000 years ago in ancient Mesopotamia (modern-day Iraq), again brought with it erotic (or pornographic) expression, such as this extract from "The Courtship of Inanna and Dumuzi", one of the world's oldest known love poems:

Inanna spoke:
"My vulva, the horn,
The Boat of Heaven,
Is full of eagerness like the young moon.
My untilled land lies fallow.
As for me, Inanna,
Who will plow my vulva?
Who will plow my high field?

Who will plow my wet ground?
As for me, the young woman,
Who will plow my vulva?
Who will station the ox there?
Who will plow my vulva?"

Dumuzi replied:
"Great Lady, the king will plow your vulva?
I, Dumuzi the King, will plow your vulva."
Inanna:
"Then plow my vulva, man of my heart!
Plow my vulva!"
...
The shepherd Dumuzi filled my lap with cream and milk,
He stroked my pubic hair,
He watered my womb.
He laid his hands on my holy vulva,
He smoothed my black boat with cream,
He quickened my narrow boat with milk,
He caressed me on the bed.[1]

This poem would be censored in many modern societies, including some that consider themselves liberal bastions of free speech. It might be labelled as ungodly, permissive, obscene, harmful to children or offensive to women. In some ways, we don't appear to have come very far in the past 5000 years.

The Eternal Backlash against Sexual Expression

The sexual art from ancient societies reveals our eternal obsession with sex, and also a second aspect of human sexual history: societies appear to go through cycles of sexual freedom followed by repression. It seems that each leap forward in the open expression and discussion of sexuality is later met with a backlash, with the intent of pushing sexual expression back underground. As notable as the appearance of overtly sexual Venus figures across a wide area of prehistoric Europe, Asia and Africa, is the fact of their vanishing. History and prehistory appear to be dotted with a series of sexual revolutions, each one ending with a backlash and a rise in conservative, anti-sex attitudes. Perhaps the only thing as universal in human society as a love of sex is a fear of sex, and history witnesses a never-ending tussle between these two great forces.

Just as writing brought about new forms of highly sexual expression in Mesopotamia, it was later seized upon as a tool to bring about the rise of religious power, and with it political control. The Middle East, being the birthplace of civilisation and of writing, inevitably became the source of many of the world's great religions. The Old and New Testaments of the Bible, written over the course of around 1600 years of turbulent Middle Eastern history, demonstrate the evolution of sexual morality. A state machine was emerging, with the holy texts as the source of its power, and unlike the earlier Mesopotamian celebration of sex, Biblical attitudes to sexuality are often repressive ones. Over time, sex gradually becomes acceptable only within marriage, or sometimes as a prize to soldiers for military conquest.

The rise and fall of sexual freedoms, including explicit sexual expression, appears to march hand in hand with the rise and fall of political freedoms. Lenin's Soviet Union, in its post-revolutionary burst of exuberant liberty, was the first modern state to decriminalise homosexuality; but as the nation lapsed swiftly back into authoritarian dictatorship, Stalin re-criminalised it in 1933, and homosexual behaviour remained underground for another 60 years, until post-Soviet Russia experienced another, brief, upsurge in political and social liberty in the 1990s. Nazi Germany attacked and criminalised sexual expression, homosexuality and abortion rights. The Vatican was a powerful supporter of Italian fascism, the Franco dictatorship in Spain, and US-backed dictatorships in Latin America, and all of these repressive regimes were marked with a rise in support for 'family values', and intolerance for sexual expression, women's reproductive rights and homosexuality.

The 1950s McCarthy era in the United States was perhaps America's greatest deviation away from its founding principle of free speech, as communists (or to be more accurate, people labelled communists) were attacked and suppressed. Unsurprisingly, McCarthy's Red Scare was also accompanied by a strengthening in anti-sex 'family values', and a lesser-known witch-hunt against homosexuals known as the Lavender Scare.

In a 1993 *Playboy* article, the writer Peter Hamill wrote about the link between sexual and political freedoms:

> Recent history teaches us that most tyrannies have a puritanical nature. The sexual restrictions of Stalin's Soviet Union, Hitler's Germany and Mao's China would have gladdened the hearts of those Americans who fear sexual images and literature. Their ironfisted puritanism wasn't motivated by a need to erase inequality. They wanted to smother the personal chaos that can accompany sexual freedom and subordinate it to the granite face of the state. Every tyrant knows that if he can control human sexuality, he can control life.[2]

So, political and sexual freedoms appear to be inseparable, though cause and effect are harder to identify. Often, sexual expression is the first form of expression to come under attack by a repressive state machine, simply because it represents the softest target; it is easier to convince a frightened public that pornography, nudity and erotic art are somehow harmful than it is to openly attack free speech. But once censorship mechanisms are established, once populations accept the role of the censor as a valid one, all forms of expression can, and will, come under attack. Societies that are intolerant of free speech will be particularly intolerant of any expression related to minorities, including sexual minorities. Social conservatives – those people who most strongly believe that human nature must be regulated and controlled – are the very people most likely to thrive under authoritarian political regimes, and to be appointed to censorship roles.

Where Are We Now?

So if attacks on sexual expression are a proxy for rising intolerance and authoritarianism in general, one can quickly gauge the current state of a society by watching its anti-porn campaigners, examining how seriously they are taken by the mass media and politicians, and measuring the effectiveness of their banning campaigns. One can also examine the attitudes of the next generation of adults: student attitudes, above all, are a good proxy for the state of society now and in the near future. Universities are traditionally thought of as places of tolerance, intelligence and free thought; if a subject cannot be intelligently and politely discussed on campus, where can it be?

On this basis, we have something to fear. For example, some student unions have recently voted to ban the widely disliked, but still popular, *Sun* newspaper from university campuses, primarily on the basis that topless women can be seen on Page 3. This comes in spite of the fact that the paper's circulation has been in decline for years (as have those of most paper publications), that Page 3 has been a daily feature for over four decades, and that – unlike in 1973 when Page 3 was born – images of topless women can now easily be found online. In other words, such bans come not in response to a rising new threat, but as an exercise in authoritarian muscle-flexing.

The censorship effect of banning a newspaper on campus is almost insignificant in practice, but what it signals is deeply disturbing. A new generation of students has seized on censorship as an acceptable tool with which to further political or moral goals, and this extends far beyond the *Sun*. They ban it because they can, because they enjoy the power that censorship brings, and because tolerance for other people's 'unacceptable' reading habits has apparently fizzled away on university campuses. We might note that the *Sun* has a primarily working-class readership, and university student unions are pretty middle-class affairs. The stench of snobbery and class bullying can often be detected where censorship is involved: elitists have rarely doubted their right to judge and control the reading matter of the lower classes.

Today's advocates for censorship are not necessarily opposed to sexual expression. When I founded the Sex & Censorship campaign and blog in 2013, I attracted many supporters who identified as pro-porn and sex-positive, and assumed that such people must also be anti-censorship. As my blogging progressed, I found that many apparently liberal people were only opposed to censorship of things they enjoyed, but would not extend that principle to things they disapproved of. So, for example, there was the young woman who enthusiastically backed my opposition to the government ban on 'rape porn', but who believed Page 3 should be removed from the *Sun*. There was the sex blogger who often retweeted my pro-pornography links, but became apoplectic when I flagged concern about a moral panic taking place against (allegedly) misogynistic computer games. Campaigning against censorship on principle, it turned out, can be a lonely business.

Is it Censorship?

Almost nobody ever proudly proclaims themselves to be pro-censorship. This is especially true in today's climate, when some of the most ardent advocates of censorship are to the left of centre and see themselves as pretty liberal types. Dictionary.com provides five definitions of 'censor', of which the first two are useful for the purposes of this book. The first is the one that most people would think of:

An official who examines books, plays, news reports, motion pictures, radio and television programs, letters, cablegrams, etc., for the purpose of suppressing parts deemed objectionable on moral, political, military, or other grounds.

But it is important to understand that censorship is something that *anybody* can do, and the more social power a person has, the more they can censor. The second, more useful definition is:

Any person who supervises the manners or morality of others.

This applies, for example, to those student-union committee members that vote to ban the *Sun* from being sold on campus. Getting oneself elected to the student union brings a little bit of power to control the flow of information. But in this digital age, it can apply equally well to anyone. The Internet has democratised publishing, and pushed the power of disseminating information down to the masses. Today, we are all publishers (if we choose), as well as readers, and we all pick and choose what to publish.

As soon as a person opens a Twitter or Facebook account, they are at liberty to begin censoring their own view of the world, simply by following people they like and blocking people they dislike. At the individual level, it is hard to argue that this is in any way harmful: even I have occasionally blocked people that persist in tweeting abuse at me. But on a mass scale, this form of censorship might be one of the most corrosive.

Much has been written recently on the creation of 'echo chambers' – clusters of people on social media that deliberately censor their view of the world by only listening to people they agree with anyway. Worrying research has found that, increasingly, people choose not to listen to anything they dislike or disagree with. One recent piece of research[3] analysed online debates about climate change, and found that almost no commentator was being listened to by both sides. I was named in the research (or rather @MoronWatch, a political Twitter account I run, was named) as one of very few people that was being followed by both sides. This was personally gratifying, but also depressing. Rather than convince deniers that climate change requires action, commentators are increasingly shouting, pointlessly, at the converted.

Similarly, I have witnessed some of my left-wing Facebook friends boasting that they unfriended people, whether for opposing gay marriage, voting Tory or some other form of thought crime. This behaviour puzzles me: my aim in conducting political discourse is to change minds, not to hide from unpalatable ideas. Instead of joyously using our newfound power to challenge views we dislike, some of us prefer instead to pretend we live in a perfect world where nobody disagrees with us. A medium that has united humankind globally is also segregating us: this could prove dangerous.

So censorship is any act that disrupts the free flow of information, from a ban on reporting a particular story, to the murder of a blogger. While the most powerful acts of censorship are carried out by state machines, increasingly censorship is becoming an activity that anyone can do. For those of us that celebrated the unprecedented freedom of expression brought about by the Internet, this has been an unexpected development.

Moral panics, the core subject of this book, are designed to make censorship and other forms of repression more acceptable, by persuading the public, the media and the political class that mere expression – words, pictures, videos, ideas – can, in some way, cause harm. Moral entrepreneurs – the people who architect and drive moral panics – must move with the times. Their message must chime with a large segment of the population, and especially with the young. It is exactly because of the triumph of liberal values in the second half of the 20th century that today's highly illiberal anti-sex messages have been recrafted in the language of liberalism.

3

The Trouble with Winning

If I can't dance, I don't want your revolution! – Emma Goldman

Pondering on the fresh election of the left-winger Jeremy Corbyn as leader of the Labour Party, a friend put his finger on what made the event so exciting. "We're just so used to losing", he said. Although I was less of a Corbynite than he, I saw his point. Both of us had become involved in left-wing politics just as Thatcher and Reagan began their joint crusade to erode social democracy and shift power back to the market, a moment that turned out to be a significant historical turning point.

Over the following decade, we saw our side lose every battle it fought, and we became used to losing. Trade unions were defeated time and again, most notably during the miners' strike of 1984/5, the sad ending of which broke the morale of the labour movement. State-owned industries and assets were privatised. The huge fortresses of industrial militancy, from coal mines to steel mills, were closed down or heavily automated. The industrial working class, which had brought down a Conservative government in 1974, was a shrinking, spent political force by 1990, and plummeting trade-union membership reflected this new reality. We had grown up in a world divided into nominally capitalist and socialist societies. With the collapse of the Soviet Union, and the switch of Russia and Eastern Europe to a market-based economy (China having begun similar reforms in 1979), the global left, a series of movements dating back to the mid-19th century, appeared to have run out of steam.

The 1980s was a dismal time to be on the left, and unsurprisingly, many activists drifted away. What remained of the political left was no longer based in heavy industry, in working-class towns and inner cities, or among immigrant populations; instead it increasingly retrenched within public-service unions and sections of academia. It became more middle-class and whiter, subtly adopted new values, and began to evolve into a very different movement.

Historically, the left had tended to be aligned with socially liberal values, and the right with conservative ones, although these links were never absolute. Before discussing the parting of ways between liberal values and the new left, it is worth reminding ourselves where these movements originated.

Liberalism and the Left

The Enlightenment refers to a broad political and philosophical movement that appeared in Western Europe during the 18th century. It was spurred by the young science revolution, and held the triumph of reason over superstition to be among its core values. Liberalism emerged as the political philosophy of Enlightenment thinkers, and – other than Reason – had as its values individual Liberty and Equality for all. Liberals were suspicious of powerful government, especially at a time when government was synonymous with royalty and state-imposed religion, and liberals sought to find ways in which to limit state power.

Although much Enlightenment thought originated in Britain – and especially from the philosopher John Locke – its greatest political effects were felt in two other countries late in the 18th century: first in the United States, which threw off British rule during its revolution, and established a liberal constitution; then in France's revolution.

The success of these revolutions can be endlessly debated, and few would claim that either country, today, is a wonderful example of Enlightenment values. However, one of the most powerful lasting legacies of the Enlightenment age is the First Amendment to the US Constitution, which guarantees freedom of speech, of the press, of assembly, and of religion. This piece of text has had a fundamental influence over American culture; one of its many effects has been to establish America as the centre of a huge social revolution: the explosive rise of modern, explicit pornography.

The left was born (along with, unsurprisingly, the right) during the French revolution, and referred to the seating arrangement in the National Assembly: supporters of the revolution sat to the president's left, and monarchists to his right. Thus, the left was a product of the Enlightenment and became broadly associated with progress, and the right with maintenance of the status quo.

During the 19th century, intellectuals of the European left debated, wrote pamphlets and books, and divided into multiple strands, from anarchists to communists. The tenets of liberalism – liberty, reason, equality – were embraced to a greater or lesser extent across these various groupings. In the 20th century, clear divisions appeared between sections of the left and liberalism; most obviously the Soviet Union, and its communist supporters worldwide, rejected individual liberty. The USSR's version of equality was also suspect ("All animals are equal, but some animals are more equal than others", wrote Orwell in *Animal Farm*).

However, in the West, the mainstream left remained a broadly liberal force, at least until the 1970s.

What Do You Do after You've Won?

In a historical context, the left's big problem by the time my Corbynite friend and I became activists was that, by many measures, it had already won. The Attlee Labour government, elected by a landslide in 1945, had made real the dreams of earlier generations of socialists. Universal education and healthcare, a welfare state to defend the poorest, public ownership of key industries: these immense reforms would eradicate the worst forms of poverty that had been experienced by pre-war generations, and create the conditions for a growing, confident middle class. If Karl Marx had been propelled forward in time to the late 20th century, he would not have seen his Communist utopia brought to life, but neither would he have recognised the rapacious, uncontrolled capitalism that had inspired his Communist Manifesto.

Social democracy – a pragmatic blend of free markets, welfare states and selective state intervention – was the order of the day in Britain and Western Europe, and this new order became broadly accepted by both the mainstream left and right. The left–right divide ceased to be a deeply ideological one, and instead became a numbers game. How much should the state raise in taxes, and from whom? Which services should be state-operated, and which left to the market or charities to provide? How much regulation of business was the right amount? How broad and how strong should be the safety net that kept the poorest out of poverty?

With these economic gains won, the postwar revolution switched its sights towards new, social goals. The Labour government of the late-1960s (under the deeply liberal Home Secretary Roy Jenkins) brought forth sweeping social reform in tune with the sexual and social revolution of the day, of most significance being the abandonment of the death penalty, decriminalisation of homosexuality, divorce-law reform and the legalisation of abortion. In the early-70s, the liberalising reforms continued with the recognition of rape within marriage as a crime, the passage of the Equal Pay Act and the provision of the contraceptive pill on the National Health Service to single women (it had been available to married women since 1961). These were all key victories for the feminist movement, and the liberal left in general.

Censored UK

But perhaps Britain's Swinging Sixties had begun in earnest in 1959, when the archaic Obscene Publications Act had been overhauled, following a long campaign by Roy Jenkins, then in opposition. The OPA had formed the bedrock of British censorship law for a century, and allowed police to seize and destroy material that they believed might 'deprave and corrupt' those who viewed it. It was, in particular, an effective and draconian tool against publishers of sexual expression, though it could be used against anything the state believed to be offensive or dangerous. The liberalised Act allowed exemptions for artistic merit and public good, and so created the conditions for authors, photographers and filmmakers to begin pushing the boundaries of British censorship. The following year, Penguin Books was prosecuted for publishing *Lady Chatterley's Lover*, DH Lawrence's highly erotic novel. The prosecutor famously opened his case by asking:

Would you approve of your young sons, young daughters – because girls can read as well as boys – reading this book? Is it a book you would have lying around your own house? Is it a book that you would even wish your wife or your servants to read?

The jury responded to this laughable statement by finding Penguin not-guilty, thus demonstrating how far out of step the British establishment was with the general public. The book was published, became a bestseller and eventually a classic. This was the start of a long journey to irrelevance for the OPA. Juries would tend not to be nearly as easily offended as the British state, and so would often acquit defendants. Over the intervening years, attempted prosecutions under the OPA have steadily declined, to the point where the Act is rarely used today.

In hindsight, Jenkins might have been better advised to leave his attempts to reform the OPA until the late-1960s, when it might possibly have been scrapped altogether. In 1969, Denmark legalised pornography. Sweden followed suit in 1970 and West Germany in 1973. Britain remained saddled with an anti-pornography law that, in the climate of the late-60s and early-70s, appeared draconian and outdated.

In the late-70s, the Home Office established a Committee on Obscenity and Film Censorship (known as the Williams Committee, after its chair, Bernard Williams). The committee examined the available research on pornography, and heard testimony from the morality campaigner Mary Whitehouse. Whitehouse stated that porn was harmful, and claimed to have letters from women who had been abused within the industry; but upon her failure to produce the letters[4], her testimony was dismissed. The committee concluded in 1979 that "the role of pornography in influencing society is not very important... to think anything else is to get the problem of pornography out of proportion with the many other problems that face our society today", and recommended full legalisation for adult consumption, which would have entailed a major overhaul of obscenity law. The Williams Committee's findings were in line with a similar, US-based inquiry – the President's Commission on Obscenity and Pornography – that had been conducted a decade earlier. When the President's Commission reported it could find no solid evidence that porn was harmful, Congress had refused to accept the report.

So by the late-1970s, the core of British censorship law looked obsolete; surely it was a matter of time before the OPA was scrapped, and along with it, Britain's tight restrictions on pornography? But the political culture of Britain and much of the Western world had changed markedly since the 1960s. The great liberal era had quietly drawn to a close during the 70s, and social conservatism was beginning to gain the upper hand again. 1979 – the year the Williams Committee reported – was also the year of a general election that heralded the first big rightward swing since WWII, and the election of Margaret Thatcher as Prime Minister.

Rebuilding the Censorship State

Social conservatives must have looked on in dismay at the declining power of UK obscenity law, which had left a gaping hole in their abilities to control access to sexual and other expression that offended their sensibilities. They set out, bit by bit, to create a new censorship framework: one that left censorship decisions in the hands of professional censors rather than juries. They have been remarkably successful in doing so. Since the late-70s, the continuous trend has been towards more, then more, and then yet more censorship, introduced for multiple reasons, against a variety of targets, and implemented in many ways. This trend has proceeded uninterrupted for almost four decades, across governments of all colours. There has been no intervening liberal period similar to the Jenkins era, during which the state or politicians have questioned the need for new censorship laws, let alone rolled old ones back.

The tool for achieving ever-more censorship is the moral panic, a process in which campaigners, the media and assorted vested interests conspire to create the belief in the public mind that some vast new threat has come into being, and that Something Must Be Done. Small numbers of adept and well-connected individuals – or even just one – can work to stir up fear, via clever use of the mass media (or in more recent times, social media). Once the seeds of fear are planted, the architects – known as moral entrepreneurs – lobby politicians for some change to the law to address the stated problem. For politicians, even those who doubt the veracity of the threat, there is little to gain by opposing new censorship legislation, but much to lose. No MP would relish being the one named in the press as an apologist for some unspeakable threat to women and children.

From the 1960s until she died in 2001, the most effective British moral entrepreneur was the tireless Mary Whitehouse. In terms of creating moral panics in order to achieve changes to the British legal landscape, she was highly successful. Her first triumph came in 1978, when she utilised a powerful, and at that time unknown, concept: 'child pornography'. Although this term is widely used today, it is worth noting in passing that child-protection professionals dislike it, preferring to refer to 'child-abuse imagery'. Referring to such material as pornography creates a link in the mind of the casual observer between child rape and consenting sex between adults. This is, of course, one of the purposes of the term. To make such a comparison in most contexts would provoke a horrified response, but in the context of pornography, the term is widely used, and creates a vague impression to observers that child abuse constitutes some inevitable dark side of the porn industry. It thus helps build the bogus argument that, in order to rid the world of child abuse and other forms of sexual crime, we must expunge it of all sexual expression, even the softest forms.

Whitehouse took the template for her anti-child porn campaign from the US, where a similar moral panic had taken place, and found fertile ground in the British media. It is probably not coincidental that the first video recorder for home use was launched in 1978, feeding into the idea that Britain's island status was coming under threat from pernicious, foreign influences that had previously been held back – along with other nasty, foreign stuff – at the white cliffs of Dover.

The media enthusiastically joined the campaign for a ban on child porn, and Whitehouse's efforts were rewarded by the passage of the Protection of Children Act. However – and this is a common feature of censorship laws resulting from moral panics – the Act's effects were far broader than just to target child-abuse imagery. The wording of the law instead referred vaguely to 'indecent imagery of children'. This broad terminology would have major repercussions. In the shorter term, it led to the arrest of people, and sometimes to huge damage to their lives, for taking naked pictures of their children: something that many, if not most, parents do. The most famous of these cases was that of the TV newsreader Julia Somerville, who was arrested in 1995, along with her partner, for taking photographs of their seven-year old daughter in the bath. They were not charged, but the arrest wreaked havoc on their lives and reputations.

The law blurred the distinction between child nudity and child rape. Two entirely different things, one arguably harmless (or even healthy) and the other undoubtedly harmful, have been associated with each other. This linkage works well for the purposes of anti-sex conservatives, however, in that it stigmatises nudity as something dirty and unhealthy, reinforcing an age-old British attitude.

More recently, with the arrival of smartphones and selfie culture, the law has taken a more dangerous turn. Teenagers who have snapped and shared naked selfies – reportedly an increasingly normal aspect of teen sexuality – find themselves accused of making indecent imagery, and at threat of being charged as sex offenders. Anyone who receives such an image, even unsolicited, is again at risk of being labelled a sex offender. There have been a number of such cases: In September 2015, for example, a 14-year-old British boy was reported to have sent a naked image of himself to his girlfriend, who decided to share it more widely. The picture was later discovered and reported. Although police decided not to arrest or charge the boy, his details (and possibly those of his girlfriend and others who shared the image) were reportedly added to a police information database, where they could be held for up to ten years, and accessible to searches by future employers.

Thanks to an anomaly in the law, even consenting adults can be criminalised for sexting. Indecent imagery of children applies to any model under 18; but the age of consent in Britain is 16. This means that that a 17 year old can legally have sex, but if they photograph themselves in action, they are creating 'indecent imagery of children'.

There are other unexpected side-effects of such laws in the Internet age: anybody that casually browses mainstream online pornography sites might inadvertently be at risk of being branded a sex offender, with all that entails. Today's porn sites present a long page of thumbnail images that tempt the viewer to click further. Unless the viewer is careful to use their browser's *incognito* mode (this is named somewhat differently for each browser), the images will be cached on the device: this constitutes 'possession' in the eyes of the law. Some images might feature models that *appear* to be under 18. In the event that such an image is found on a person's phone or laptop, the police do not have to prove the model is underage, the accused must prove that he or she is 18 or more. The user may have never actually *seen* the image: it might have been at the bottom of a long page for example.

Here, there is no suggestion that the model is actually a child being abused: in fact, porn studios are required to ensure that all models they employ are over 18. Nor is there the serious possibility that the viewer in such a case is a threat to children. Yet, there is a genuine chance of being labelled one, being found guilty, being placed on the sex-offenders register, and being imprisoned or fined, with all the ramifications for the person's reputation, family life and career.

In 2011, one such case found a British man accused of accessing underage gay pornography. The Crown Prosecution Service decided to prosecute, without trying to determine the actual ages of the models; it was only thanks to the persistence of the man's legal team that the studio was traced, and model ID records obtained. Despite being provided with proof that no law had been broken, the CPS waited several more months before dropping the case. In other cases, people have been prosecuted for receiving, unsolicited, potentially illegal images via email or WhatsApp. These, and other similar cases, indicate strong official enthusiasm to brand people sex offenders on the flimsiest of evidence. A system purportedly introduced to protect children from sexual abuse has become a tool in the hands of authorities to victimise countless individuals, and stigmatise online sexual expression. While ruining some people's lives, the authorities are sending a clear message to millions: enjoy online porn at your peril.

Anti-child abuse imagery laws serve a vital purpose of child protection as well as undoubtedly having dangerous side effects. They also, in practice, affect relatively few people (though in theory, millions risk being criminalised). Following her 'child porn' moral panic, Mary Whitehouse's next campaign had a far more significant outcome, and resulted in a law which arguably serves no useful purpose, but has had long-lasting effects on British culture and law.

Video Nasties

As video recorders became cheaper, their adoption in British homes became widespread. For the first time, British film viewers could choose what to watch, regardless of the highly censorious attitudes of the authorities. Video libraries suddenly popped up on every high street to cater for a huge upsurge in demand: my first job, in the summer of 1983, was in one of these exciting new places.

Until this spread of video in the early-1980s, film releases had long been censored by a regime of local-authority licensing. Although cinemas could, in theory, show audiences whatever they chose, to show pornography, strong horror and other non-approved material could mean the withdrawal of their licenses by local authorities. To make life easier for cinema owners, the film industry had (as far back as 1912) set up its own censorship body, the British Board of Film Censors. As well as censoring films, the BBFC awarded them a certificate as an indication to cinemas and filmgoers of the type of content to be expected. A BBFC certificate was not legally binding, but it allowed cinema owners to stay safely within obscenity law. The system also ensured that, in practice, films falling foul of the BBFC's tight guidelines could not be commercially successful.

Throughout 1983 and into 1984, a moral panic over video took root, its specific target being a new brand of low-budget horror movies, often made for video, which were designed to shock. Mary Whitehouse was the lead figure in coordinating the panic, and she found enthusiastic support from a variety of powers, especially the tabloid press, senior police officers, prosecutors and the BBFC. To the latter (being a private organisation), video comprised both a threat to their business of film censorship, and an opportunity for expansion.

Termed by the tabloids 'video nasties', the new wave of horror films became blamed for every ill in society. The video nasties moral panic is perhaps the best-documented in British history, having been the subject of academic studies, books and the 2010 documentary *Video Nasties: Moral Panic, Censorship & Videotape*. Bogus statistics were employed to show that half – or even more – of children had seen such titles, and hysterical claims were made about their effects on the young psyche. Newspapers – tabloid and broadsheet alike – warned of a generation of rapists and murderers, unless the nasties could be quickly reined in.

Parliamentary lobbying by Whitehouse resulted in strong support for action by MPs of all parties, and eventually the Video Recordings Act was introduced to Parliament. The power of a successfully run moral panic was demonstrated in the lack of opposition that was raised to the Act. Despite it introducing state censorship on an almost unprecedented scale, there was no outcry from press, politicians or campaigners – at least, other than the almost-solo efforts of an academic, Martin Barker, who had found the published research to be nonsense, and bravely set out to be the bogeyman who would defend video nasties.

The Video Recordings Act came into force in 1984, and empowered the BBFC – still an unaccountable, private organisation – as the UK's official censor of video. Now, any person who distributed a video title without a BBFC certificate could be prosecuted, regardless of its content. At a stroke, the safeguards within the Obscene Publications Act were removed. Instead of a jury, it was now the BBFC that decided whether a title was obscene or not. They could refuse to issue a certificate, and any subsequent distribution of the work would automatically constitute a criminal offence, even if the BBFC's original decision was later modified.

Almost no other democratic country has implemented a system of video censorship like the one the UK has had in place since 1984. From that point onwards, British citizens had to settle for more tightly censored video works, especially in the realm of pornography.

The Quiet Porn Ban

Following the passage of the VRA, mention of video nasties fizzled away overnight. Many of the 'worst' titles cited during the moral panic have since been granted BBFC certificates, and are legally available anyway. Of far more significance was the BBFC's unilateral decision to ban hard-core pornography – a genre that was now widespread in Europe and the US – in its entirety.

It is worth reflecting on the fact that this sweeping, moralistic act of censorship was carried out without a shred of parliamentary oversight. Here was an unelected body writing government policy without any of the trappings of democracy. Nor was there any outcry questioning this decision: porn is a wonderful target for censorship, as the worthy defenders of civil liberties tend to avert their gaze when it is under attack. So it is hardly surprising that in recent years, the focus of attempts to censor the Internet has again been porn (although terrorism also makes an appearance from time to time).

Pornography had already been entirely banned from television by a patchwork of regulatory bodies. These were later merged to form the immense, powerful and unelected super-regulator, Ofcom, which, like the BBFC, writes and implements its own legal code. So from 1984 onward, UK consumers were blocked from legitimately accessing, on TV and on video, sexually explicit material that was, by now, widely and legally available across Europe.

It took almost two decades for the porn industry to success-fully challenge the BBFC's porn ban in court, and by this point, Internet porn had become widely available anyway. The British porn-DVD industry saw a boom in the early years of the new century following its legalisation, but this did not last long. A combination of industrial-scale piracy and broadband Internet connections would banish pornographic video, and its successor format DVD, back to the margins again.

The rapid uptake of video by British consumers of the early-1980s was an example of a phenomenon that would repeat with increasing intensity: apparently robust censorship regimes could be entirely side-tracked by the sudden arrival of a new and unexpected technology – and most new technologies are, more or less, unexpected. The forward march of communications technologies, from video to satellite television and then the web and streaming, served to repeatedly breach walls of censorship that had been carefully constructed to cope with existing 'threats' to public decency. For those of us opposed to most state censorship, technology has been our friend. It has not only allowed consumers to entirely ignore censorship regimes, but has helped to demonstrate that material labelled 'dangerous' by the authorities was not actually dangerous at all.

But there is a darker side to this: technology has also helped hide from the public the sheer scope of the censorship state being constructed in our country; in large part, these censors write their own rules and apply their own punishments. They are largely beyond parliamentary oversight (or at least, few politicians have shown any interest in providing oversight), and in some ways they circumvent the court system: they have created a shadow legal system. For almost four decades, a growing weight of law and regulation has been put into place, always running to catch up with technological innovation; but even the most ardent technophile must accept that the authorities, slow as they are to understand change, will eventually catch up. When they do – and the signs are that the moment is near – the power of the censors will come as a shock to a population that has become used to accessing whatever content it chooses.

Extreme Porn

When we launched Strictly Broadband in 2004, the only censorship law affecting us was the Obscene Publications Act. So long as we steered clear of obviously 'obscene' material, we were safe from prosecution. But how to decide what might be obscene? The OPA itself provides no clue, simply leaving a jury to decide whether the content is liable to 'deprave and corrupt' a typical viewer. This clearly creates problems for publishers seeking to work within the law. It is also problematic for police and prosecutors: Who to arrest? Who to charge? Who to prosecute?

The BBFC also requires guidance on which material should be cut, and which left in. For this reason, the CPS, police and BBFC have developed shared guidelines defining, in detail, their own idea of obscenity. The BBFC's R18 certificate, for pornographic material, is designed based on the obscenity guidelines, but leaves a large margin of error. In other words, the BBFC will often censor material that would not result in an obscenity prosecution – they will explain that this gap represents a 'precautionary' approach, though some might suspect it is merely censorship for the sake of censorship.

The guidelines cover acts that are considered to be harmful – whipping and fisting are examples – as well as acts that are not harmful but considered to be immoral – urination as a sexual act, for example. But even then, for publishers, where are the boundaries? The case of fisting (insertion of a hand into a vagina or anus) gives a good example of the Kafkaesque world of the censors. Fingering is allowed, but where is the line between fingering and fisting? This may seem irrelevant and arbitrary, but BBFC examiners are required to watch video, second-by-second, to determine when lines have been crossed. For material to be prosecuted for obscenity, a hand must be inserted past the wrist; but the BBFC, in its self-appointed quest to keep the British public safe from fisting, cuts content to a more conservative limit, and has informally agreed a 'four-finger rule' with the British porn industry. So long as the thumb is visible, the Board considers content safe for consumption. It is unclear whether BBFC examiners are depraved and/or corrupted by having to see obscene material during their work.

As a video-on-demand service, we had no need to submit material for certification by the BBFC, but this also left us having to make our own censorship decisions to protect ourselves. In practice, this meant that we would be more or less bold in our publishing decisions depending how brave I felt on any particular day. I would avoid the strongest sado-masochistic material, while pushing the boundaries in other areas: female ejaculation, for example, is frowned upon by the BBFC, but I did not believe this would ever result in an obscenity prosecution, so I often allowed it.

I long suspected that the authorities were quietly seething that a service like ours could largely ignore guidelines set by Ofcom (for TV) and the BBFC (for DVD), and I was right. Behind the scenes, censors were working hard on ways to rein us back in. In the absence of any way (in the short term) to block content en-masse, the authorities instead reached for draconian powers against consumers.

In 2008, the Labour government introduced Section 63 of the Criminal Justice and Immigration Act, better known as the extreme-porn law. This outlawed the possession of four categories of pornography: bestiality, necrophilia, life-threatening acts and acts that might damage genitals, anuses and breasts. The latter two categories, in practice, criminalised acts that are perfectly legal to carry out in private. Strangulation, for example, is a common sexual practice, but is deemed by the censors to be 'life-threatening'. It is legal to do, but should one record oneself doing it, one faces prosecution for extreme-porn possession. And fisting, another legal and popular sex act, also becomes a crime when recorded.

Possession laws are draconian because they place the onus on the average person to know what the bounds of legality are. Given how broad the categories are, and how vague the limits, this is basically impossible. I am one of perhaps a few thousand people in the country with a reasonable understanding of the guidelines. Ninety-nine per cent of the population has no idea that they might easily break the law, and face a prison sentence, by browsing online porn.

The broad concept of 'possession' also seems designed to entrap people. In one of the highest-profile extreme-porn cases, that of Simon Walsh, the prosecution was based on images (of gay anal fisting) that had been sent to his Hotmail account. The images came from a party that Walsh himself had attended. He could call the 'victims' as witnesses to demonstrate that their anuses had definitely not been harmed by the act; but this was not a defence against online pornography – he had to prove that the act could *never* be harmful. Walsh was eventually found not-guilty by a jury, but his finances had been ruined, and his political and legal career shattered.

In another well-known case – the Tiger Porn Trial – a Welsh man was prosecuted for possessing a computer-generated video of a woman having sex with a tiger. The case reached court, before being thrown out as obviously ludicrous. The man had temporarily lost access to his children, and had been assaulted and abused in his hometown, as the result of being charged with a 'serious sexual offence'. Since the Act was passed, thousands of people have pleaded guilty to extreme-porn possession rather than face the publicity of a trial or the risk of jail.

Just as with the harassment of teens for sexting, the only obvious outcome of the extreme-porn law has been to send the signal that browsing and sharing sexual imagery is unacceptable in the eyes of the British state. In particular, the law has crimi- nalised the sex lives of fetishists, who often engage – perfectly legally – in many acts that they are no longer allowed to record or watch.

From a distance, the extreme-porn law looks like nothing more than the vicious lashing-out of a state that was losing its ability to prevent people enjoying and recording varied, adven- turous sex lives. It was a response to the fact that the OPA cannot be used against foreign distributors of online porn, and to the fact that, anyway, British juries appear to have little appetite for prosecuting people for obscenity.

The extreme-porn law was really a stop-gap. What the authorities really wanted was to directly control the flow of content online by the technical ability to block, en-masse, access to millions of websites. In other words, the censors' dream has been to introduce a system of direct Internet censorship akin to that in China.

The Audiovisual Media Services Directive

The vehicle being used to create the first state Internet censor in the democratic world is an innocuous EU directive known as the Audiovisual Media Services Directive, AVMS, which came into effect in 2010.

Although the EU's intention was merely to extend existing

broadcast rules to new, competing VoD services (such as iPlayer and Netflix), British regulators seized on the directive as a tool for censoring online pornography. Thus, alone in the EU, Britain introduced a new (and expensive) regulator to implement AVMS: ATVOD, the Authority for Television on Demand.

ATVOD, like the BBFC, was a private organisation, to which Ofcom had delegated its powers. This meant that ATVOD could accuse providers of breaching its rules, and then pass the case to Ofcom, which could impose fines of up to £250,000. The scale of these punishments is immense; sanctions that were originally introduced to regulate broadcasting corporations were now being deployed against small businesses. Although ATVOD was, in theory, supposed to regulate all VoD, it became obsessed with porn. In particular, it devoted a high proportion of its efforts to chasing down one-woman businesses: dominatrices, many of whom closed their websites rather than face enormous fines, as well as adverse publicity (ATVOD insisted on publishing the real names and addresses of 'offenders' in its determinations).

ATVOD's rules were written in-house, so as with Ofcom and the BBFC, an unelected organisation was creating and implementing public policy without democratic oversight. The crux of ATVOD's war on porn was captured in its Rule 11: a requirement to verify the ages of all visitors before they could see any sexual imagery. While this might sound reasonable at first glance, the rule was effectively impossible for any business to implement, while staying afloat. ATVOD's crusade resulted in dozens of British-based sites closing their doors, or relocating to other parts of Europe or North America.

Although ATVOD claimed its rules were designed to protect children, there was no change from a consumer perspective. Since at least 99% of the world's pornography was served from outside the UK, the regulator had no noticeable effect on anything. However, it maintained a rolling lobbying campaign for more powers (for itself) that can be summarised as: "Dear

Government, We tried to protect children from porn and everyone ignored us. Please send help!" All of this ignored the fact that parental-control filters for computers, tablets and smartphones were widely available, and had been for many years.

The central problem with ATVOD's approach was that countless millions of websites providing porn, erotica and other 'adult' content were available worldwide, and always would be. Therefore, without a state-approved censor with the power to create a UK-wide blacklist of websites, ATVOD's regulations were ineffective to the point of worthlessness. Legal changes would be needed to give the regulators any real power.

In December 2014, ATVOD's Rule 11 was quietly snuck into law by the Department of Culture Media and Sport, using a technical device known as a Statutory Instrument. Without any parliamentary discussion or vote, a law known as AVMS 2014 came into force. Now, anyone ignoring ATVOD's age-verification requirement was not just in breach of an obscure regulation, but breaking the law. In its lobbying activity, ATVOD could now make the claim that millions of websites around the globe were breaking British law. In fact, as of December 2014, well over 99 per cent of all the world's porn sites were now technically illegal in the UK. As a headline, this certainly had shock value, and could well serve to panic politicians into passing a law that would create a state-approved Internet censor.

A secondary effect of AVMS 2014 was to ban any material stronger than R18 from any British website, thus bringing the BBFC's prurient but dying censorship regime back to life. At a stroke, many fetish sites – even those that had conformed to ATVOD's age-verification requirement – were illegal. Some, which had mistakenly tried to work within British law rather than relocate, closed down at midnight the day before the law was implemented. This announcement was met with a 'face-sitting' protest outside Parliament by sexual freedom campaigners: face-sitting being one of the acts that was now banned from British websites. The protest attracted global media coverage, and global ridicule of British censorship law, but no change in the attitude of the authorities. The Liberal Democrat MP Julian Huppert – one of a handful of Commons defenders of free expression – attempted to halt the law in Parliament, but there was almost no anti-censorship appetite among his fellow MPs, and he failed.

At the time of writing (late-2015), there have been several attempts by private members to introduce an 'ATVOD law' that would empower Ofcom to block countless 'adult' websites without the need for court orders; none have so far been successful. Another attempt, known as the Online Safety Bill, is currently in process through the House of Lords.

In the autumn of 2015, it was announced that ATVOD would be dissolved, and its powers taken over by Ofcom, from the start of 2016. While this resulted in cheers from many who had come to resent ATVOD's blatantly moralistic censorship activities, it may not bode well for the future of Internet freedom (the detailed story of ATVOD's War on Porn, Britain's anti-porn censorship laws and regulations, and the drive towards Internet censorship is covered in my book *Censored UK*, to follow *Porn Panic!*)

Porn Panic!

The new laws outlined above, and others, were all aided and abetted in their passage by moral panics, orchestrated by morality campaigners and supported by bodies with vested interests in ending Internet freedom. The video-nasties moral panic of 1983/4 had taken over a year to come to fruition. Now, moral entrepreneurs had become adept at churning out one panic after another, each apparently a spontaneous response to sexual imagery in some context, but all generated by small numbers of activists.

As well as the creation of new laws, these panics were aimed at attacking sexual expression at street level. Councils were lobbied to close down strip clubs by withdrawing their licenses to trade. Supermarkets were picketed with the aim of removing lads' mags from sale. The *Sun* newspaper was implored to end Page 3. 'Black feminist' organisations popped up from nowhere, demanded censorship of 'racist, sexualised' music videos, and fizzled away again. Allegedly 'sexualised' or 'sexist' advertising could be banned based on a single complaint from a member of the public.

Mary Whitehouse, watching from heaven, has, I am confident, been applauding these new efforts to continue her work. But these new campaigners were not made in Whitehouse's image. These were left-wing groups, wielding the language of liberalism, feminism, socialism and trade-unionism to achieve goals very different from those of the old left.

In the 1930s, Europe had been swept by a wave of counter-Enlightenment, in the form of right-wing fascism. This movement had sought to bury the gains of the Enlightenment: Liberty, Equality and Reason. Fascism had posed an existential threat to Europe's liberal values, and the left had responded by declaring an all-out war against fascism. In recent years, a new counter-Enlightenment has arisen in West. While veteran anti-fascists – myself included – have spent our lives watching carefully for a resurgence of the far-right, much of this counter-Enlightenment has come from the new left. Whether we refer to these new movements as fascism, or not, is to play with semantics. The fact is, however, that sections of the left today are pursuing goals that were once the goals of fascists and of the Christian right.

This is not to say that familiar, xenophobic, far-right fascism has ceased to be a threat, and it is certainly showing a worrying resurgence in its old European strongholds, from France to Hungary, as well as rearing its head in less-expected parts of the continent, such as Scandinavia. But the end destination is more important than the route travelled. If populations accept the right of the state to intervene in the most trivial matters of inter-personal speech and political or artistic expression, it barely matters exactly *how* the state becomes empowered.

The new left's war on free expression goes far beyond a hatred of sexual expression. Censorship has become fashionable in countless contexts. This new, authoritarian, puritanical movement of the left has been so successful that the conservative right has abandoned its old moralistic language and appropriated the new terminology of the left. From left to right of the political spectrum, it has become accepted that too much free speech is a bad thing. Liberalism as a political force is at its lowest ebb in generations.

The transformation of the left from defender of the Enlightenment to protagonist of the counter-Enlightenment has taken decades. We can begin the story of this journey almost 40 years ago, in the American feminist movement.

4

How Anti-Sex Feminism Was Born

The changing names of feminist organisations tell the story. Early on, there was Women Against Violence Against Women; then, later, Women Against Violence and Pornography in the Media; and then Women Against Pornography – Marcia Pally, writer and academic

University College London (UCL) debating society is hosting a debate on the topic: "Should pornography be banned?" I am one of the four speakers, and the discussion has been opened up to contributions from the floor. A young man stands up. "I am a feminist", he says, "and therefore I am opposed to pornography". He makes a couple of points and sits down again.

At best, the contributor is guilty of intellectual laziness. He has decided to pledge allegiance to a tribe – feminists – and has therefore adopted, wholesale, what he believes to be the ideas of that tribe. Feminists (he thinks) are necessarily opposed to pornography, and since he identifies as a feminist, he too must be opposed to pornography. Tribal thinking is widespread across the political spectrum. Choosing a group to belong to saves the effort of actually having to think for oneself on a wide variety of topics.

But the speaker was guilty of more than just laziness. If he had studied the very feminist movement he claimed to follow, he would have discovered that automatic opposition to sexual expression is not an inherent aspect of feminist thought at all.

Born in the mid-1960s into a suburban London household, I was surrounded by feminist ideas from a young age. The second-wave feminist (Women's Lib) movement was in full swing during my early childhood, and my mother and her friends were typical of the women who were attracted to feminist ideas. While the first-wave feminism of the late-19th and early-20th centuries had focused on the most blatant and concrete gender inequalities in the law – notably the rights of women to vote and own property – second-wave feminism consisted of a more amorphous set of both political and cultural ideas.

The movement did have some concrete goals and demands – equal pay in the workplace, and the recognition of rape within marriage as a crime, for example – but more than that, it brought new cultural developments. While it had become normal for working-class women to work, following World War II, middle-class women were still expected to fulfil traditional female stereo-types as wives, mothers and homemakers. Women's Libbers were rebelling, not just against a state with sexist laws and attitudes, but against their own husbands and fathers.

Sexual liberation was central to the Women's Lib movement. Traditionally, women were not supposed to be creatures of lust; such behaviour was reserved for men. Female sexuality was meant to be soft, delicate and demure. Women who openly enjoyed casual sex were stigmatised as sluts. Men could sleep around, and even be admired for it, but women could not. Changing those deeply held cultural attitudes – among both men and women – was a far more challenging goal than the simple changing of laws.

Some of the defining literature of the second-wave feminist era was designed to blow away myths about female sexuality, and play a part in the sexual liberation of women. Germaine Greer's polemic *The Female Eunuch*, and the Erica Jong novel *Fear of Flying*, were each part of a cultural revolution that brought about the acceptance not just of a woman's right to be a sexual being, but that women were even capable of being such a thing.

This is not to say that second-wave feminists were all comfortable with explicit sexual expression; but in fighting for the right of women to regain control of their bodies, the movement unleashed a new generation of women who were less fearful about nudity and overt feminine sexuality. Today's army of strippers, nude models, webcam girls and pornstars, who feel no shame in baring their bodies to strangers, owe much to the Women's Lib movement. Perhaps few of today's models realise that the way they make their living today would have been considered a revolutionary act a few decades ago.

As the 70s progressed, the revolutionary fervour of the 1960s faded, and conservatism retrenched and began to mount a fightback against the new permissiveness. Conservatism was not just a force that attacked progressive movements from outside: the feminist movement itself became more conservative, in tune with the changing times. The emphasis shifted, first subtly, and then less so, away from a woman's rights over her own body and sexuality, towards a position in which sex was labelled a tool of male oppression; and thus, where sexual expression was seen as inherently oppressive towards women. By the end of the 1970s, sections of the feminist movement were markedly more socially conservative than the feminists of a decade earlier.

Tuppy Owens is a remarkable woman, who has been a publisher of erotica and a sexual-freedom campaigner since the 1960s, and runs a charity called *Outsiders*, which campaigns for the rights of disabled people to enjoy fulfilling sex lives. She recalls her first encounters with conservative feminism:

I started the Outsiders Club in 1979 for disabled men and women to gain confidence and find partners. The feminists immediately started attacking me, accusing me of encouraging disabled men to be as disgusting as other men. I can remember them sitting in their dungarees in the front row at conferences I spoke at, hurling abuse. I chose to ignore them.

For 25 years of my life, I published the Sex Maniac's Diary, a jovial pocket book with sex positions of the day, kinks of the week, and international listings of sexy hotels, swing clubs, fetish clubs and places to enjoy commercial sex. Most people bought it as a joke Christmas present but the joke was how very seriously I researched and presented the information, treating the material like it appeared in, for example, the yachting diary.

There were obviously more commercial [sex] establishments for men (as there still are), in fact hardly any for women, but the feminists decided the little diary was "sexist" and slowly printers refused to print it and criticism abounded. The charm and innocence was lost. I was very upset, but there was nothing I could do, anti-sex feminism was 'in'.[5]

The feminist movement, which began as a force for female liberation, was becoming a powerful force for censorship. In fact, as the influence of traditional, religious conservatives declined (in Britain at least, if not in the United States), anti-sex feminism took over from the religious right as *the* driving force for the censorship of sexual expression.

As with second-wave feminism itself, this conservative shift within the movement began in the United States. In 1995, the President of the American Civil Liberties Union (ACLU), Nadine Strossen, published *Defending Pornography*, a book written largely in response to the rise of what she labelled 'procensorship feminism'. In the introduction she writes on the changing nature of the anti-pornography movement:

> The startling new development is that, since the late 1970s, the traditional conservative and fundamentalist advocates of tighter legal restrictions on sexual expression have been joined by an increasingly vocal and influential segment of the feminist movement. Both groups target the sexual material they would like to curb with the pejorative label "pornography". Led by Michigan law professor Catharine MacKinnon and writer Andrea Dworkin, this faction of feminists – which

I call "MacDworkinites" – argues that pornography should be suppressed because it leads to discrimination and violence against women. Indeed, MacKinnon and Dworkin have maintained that somehow pornography itself *is* discrimination and violence against women; that its mere existence hurts women, even if it cannot be shown to cause some tangible harm.[6]

What is remarkable is that this feminist niche, led by two highly driven American activists, has come to dominate the public face of feminism in the UK as well as internationally. Furthermore, by making censorship acceptable outside of traditional conservative circles, it has helped undermine support for free expression on the political left. It is in large part thanks to the influence of Catharine MacKinnon and Andrea Dworkin that, today, a London student can state in full confidence: "I am a feminist, and therefore I am opposed to pornography".

The MacDworkinites

Anti-pornography feminism was the creation of an alliance between two women, the lawyer Catharine MacKinnon, and the political activist Andrea Dworkin. Both women expressed deep hostility not just to sexual expression, but to sexuality itself, leading some commentators to label their brand of ideology as 'anti-sex feminism'. Nadine Strossen points out:

> While the procensorship feminists' negative, traditional attitudes towards sex are on one level ironic... on another level, these attitudes are completely expected. After all, it should not be surprising that advocates of banning sexual expression would view sexuality itself with suspicion.[7]

The same applies to the anti-sex feminists I regularly encounter in debates today. Although they eschew the 'anti-sex' label, preferring 'anti-pornography', it is common to find anti-porn campaigners also fighting to ban strip clubs, prostitution and the softest forms of sexual imagery in mainstream media.

Andrea Dworkin was a left-wing firebrand, active in a number of the key progressive causes of the day, from opposing the Vietnam War to supporting abortion rights. However, on the subject of sexual expression, Dworkin departed from the permissive ideas that were prevalent on the left, and instead embraced a puritanical, anti-sex zeal more commonly associated (at that time) with religious conservatives.

Dworkin's writings on sex are explicit and disturbing, and focus on sex – including gay sex – as an act of male aggression. In her book *Pornography: Men Possessing Women*, she says: "Fucking requires that the male act on one who has less power... the one who is fucked is stigmatised as feminine during the act even when not anatomically female".[8] In her later book, *Intercourse*, Dworkin extended her analysis of pornography to all sex: "Intercourse is the pure, sterile, formal expression of men's contempt for women". Even in reference to a clothed photograph of the author Ntozake Shange, which revealed her bare shoulders, Dworkin wrote: "It's very hard to look at a picture of a woman's body and not see it with the perception that her body is being exploited".[9]

By contrast, Catharine MacKinnon was a lawyer and activist, and the daughter of George MacKinnon, a federal judge, who had served as a US Congressman. Despite her later popularity among sections of the left, she came from deeply conservative roots. Her father had been a right-wing Republican and friend of President Nixon, who had appointed him to the United States Court of Appeals, District of Columbia Circuit, in 1969.

During the 1950s McCarthyite clampdown on the political left, the American right also used the opportunity to attack other sections of society that they felt undermined 'Christian family values'. Parallel to the witch-hunts of the McCarthyite Red Scare, a lesser known Lavender Scare was underway, with homosexuals as the target; just as suspected communists were persecuted and forced out of influential positions, so were suspected gay people. As a Congressman, George MacKinnon was a protagonist of this persecution, arguing passionately in 1948 for the introduction of a 'sexual psychopath' law that would be used to target sexual minorities, primarily homosexuals. When Dr Benjamin Karpman, a psychiatrist, warned Congress that the law would criminalise a large section of American society, MacKinnon spoke up. The exchange is documented:

> When [Karpman] recommended that Washington follow the example of Europe and decriminalise private homosexual acts, Congressman MacKinnon objected. 'If there is anything I consider despicable, it is where a [homosexual] is left to prey on society.' Mackinnon drew on his own experiences in the Navy during World War II to argue that homosexual acts were often not consensual. 'They go around and they may not use actual force, but they intimidate by superior rank,' he noted. Beyond policing behaviour, such government officials wanted to contain the increasing openness, even arrogance of homosexuals.[10]

Growing up amidst such attitudes, Catharine MacKinnon's attitudes towards sex, as well as her belief that politics and the law might be used to attack sexuality, perhaps become easier to understand. According to Strossen, MacKinnon's own attitudes to sex closely mirror Dworkin's:[11]

> Catharine MacKinnon's writings offer ample variations on this same antisex theme. According to MacKinnon, feminism "sees sexuality as a social sphere of male power of which forced sex is paradigmatic." Her observations about hetero-sexual intercourse include the following: "If there is no

inequality, no violation, no dominance, no force, there is no sexual arousal"... "[T]hey just want to hurt us, dominate us and control us, and that is fucking us."

The Meese Commission: Sexual McCarthyism

Ronald Reagan's victory in the 1980 Presidential Election seemed to officially mark the death knell of the liberal era that had been born in the late-60s. There could be little doubt now that socially conservative values were back in fashion – especially since Reagan's campaign had successfully harnessed the support of a new force in US politics, the religious right, led by popular, charismatic preachers such as the televangelist Jerry Falwell.

Reagan owed favours to his Christian backers, and one of these was the creation of a new commission, set up by the Attorney General, Edwin Meese, to study the effects of pornography on society (the failure of the earlier President's Commission on Obscenity and Pornography to identify harm had outraged the right). Law professor Anthony D'Amato wrote about this new commission:

> My own interest in the rape-pornography question began in 1970 when I served as a consultant to President Nixon's Commission on Obscenity and Pornography. The Commission concluded that there was no causal relationship between exposure to sexually explicit materials and delinquent or criminal behavior. The President was furious when he learned of the conclusion. Later President Reagan tried the same thing, except unlike his predecessor he packed the Commission with persons who passed his ideological litmus test.[12]

Another professor of law, Edward de Grazia, remarked:

> The Meese Commission trundled out a parade of born-again basket-cases, antisex feminists and fun-hating fundamentalists.

Their testimony was sad, misdirected – even pathetic. It was also inflammatory, misinformed scapegoating. In a court of law such witnesses would be dismissed for lack of credibility. Trial by headline – unsupported by evidence – is a far cry from due process. But it was the method of the Meese Commission, with its fundamentalist foundation, as it had been for Joe McCarthy. This was nothing more nor less than sexual McCarthyism.[13]

Regardless of this blatant bias in the Commission's make-up, the anti-porn movement now had an apparently solid foundation on which to take its campaigns forward. There may still have been no evidence that pornography was harmful, but the Meese Report claimed it was harmful anyway, and that provided a powerful weapon in the propaganda war. The MacDworkinites were, of course, involved with the process. Dworkin gave testimony to the Commission, which featured in its final 1986 report, and Dworkin and MacKinnon held a press conference upon publication of the report.

The Meese Commission was just one of the Reagan administration's attempts to turn back the clock on sexual freedom and women's rights. The willingness of Dworkin to provide support to the administration, and give it credibility outside of its right-wing Christian base, was among the causes of a great split in the feminist movement, which is widely seen as marking the end of second-wave feminism.

Feminist Sex Wars

The arrival of anti-porn feminism led to a reaction from other feminists, who took a stand against censorship and in favour of sexual freedom and sexual expression. Thus, sex-positive feminism was born, and the feminist movement divided deeply and bitterly over the complex issues around sex, sexuality, sexual expression and censorship. This debate dominated feminist discussion during the 1980s.

There was suspicion among sex-positive feminists about the bizarre alliances created by the MacDworkinites with right-wing Christian conservatives who, in any other way, were opposed to feminism and its goals, and were rightly seen by many feminists as the enemies of women's rights. Feminist and anarchist Wendy McElroy wrote in 1984:

> There is an unholy alliance being established in this country between the moral majority and radical feminists, both of whom wish to censor pornography. [Televangelist Jerry] Falwell advocates censorship because pornography is immoral; feminists advocate censorship because pornography degrades women and provides inspiration for rapists.[14]

Anti-sex feminism necessarily painted women who appeared in pornography as helpless victims. But to make this claim, they had to attack a fundamental tenet of feminism: the importance of consent in all matters sexual. Now they were claiming that a woman could never consent to appear in pornography; they were implying that unlike men, but like children, women were incapable of making such choices for themselves.

This infantilisation of women by anti-porn feminists appeared to undermine the key things that second-wave feminism had fought for: female autonomy, and equal rights. Because all porn was considered to be abusive, women could have no right to agree to participate. Of this attitude, the author Sallie Tisdale wrote[15]:

> What a misogynistic worldview this is, this claim that women who make such choices cannot be making free choices at all… Feminists against pornography have done a sad and awful thing: They have made women into objects.

Many feminists, including many who opposed pornography, lamented the pro-censorship position as a setback for women.

Having spent years arguing that women were equally capable to men, now they saw feminists arguing that women were indeed the weaker sex, requiring additional protection from the state. Feminists For Free Expression stated[16]:

> It is ironic that just as women are finally making inroads into such male-exclusive venues as handling a skyscraper construction crane, a hostile corporate takeover attempt, and an Air Force fighter plane, we are being told that we cannot handle dirty pictures, and certainly that we would never enjoy them.

Both Dworkin and MacKinnon repeatedly demonstrated that they were strong believers in censorship, and not just to attack pornography. They also attempted to censor feminists who disagreed with them. Strossen writes that they:

> played key roles in situations involving the suppression of speech by feminist women, on issues of vital importance to women, including reproductive options and female sexuality … During the fall of 1992, Andrea Dworkin sought to prevent the publication, distribution and sale of a book about women's reproductive health, written by two respected feminists, because she disagreed with one point they made in two paragraphs of the book. Moreover, although Dworkin complained to the book's (male) publisher and orchestrated a nationwide protest and boycott effort against the book, she refused to speak to the female, feminist authors of the book, or even answer their letters.[17]

MacKinnon censored debates about pornography by refusing to share a platform with Strossen and other feminist opponents. She often succeeded in this approach, being invited to speak at universities with no opposing voices being heard, and thus strengthening the idea among those who heard her that she spoke on behalf of the feminist movement as a whole.

The Exploitation of Linda Lovelace

The story of Linda Marchiano (better known as the pornstar Linda Lovelace) has been widely told, most recently in the 2013 film *Lovelace*. Her first husband, Chuck Traynor, was controlling, violently abusive, forced her into prostitution, and coerced her into the starring role in the film that is probably the best-known porn production ever made: *Deep Throat*, made in 1972. She later divorced Traynor and married Larry Marchiano.

The publication of Marchiano's autobiography, *Ordeal*, in 1980, attracted the attention of anti-pornography feminists including Andrea Dworkin, and she became, for a while, a spokesperson for the feminist anti-pornography movement.

Dworkin and MacKinnon had the victim they needed to demonstrate the barbarity of the porn industry. And yet, Marchiano's abusive husband was not a pornographer. Her experience at his hands was an undoubtedly horrendous one, in which he frequently beat her, raped her and threatened her with guns; but she was a victim of domestic violence, not of porn-industry violence. Her experience constituted not a typical story of abuse as suffered by other women working in the industry, but a story of abuse as experienced by too many women from their partners.

She later appears to have become disenchanted with the activists:

Between Andrea Dworkin and Kitty MacKinnon, they've written so many books, and they mention my name and all that, but financially they've never helped me out. When I showed up with them for speaking engagements, I'd always get five hundred dollars or so. But I know they made a few bucks off me, just like everybody else.[18]

Despite these disagreements, Marchiano proved useful to the MacDworkinites, who needed a female victim in order to promote a legal tool they developed with which to attack pornography: the Antipornography Civil Rights Ordinance.

The Dworkin-MacKinnon Antipornography Civil Rights Ordinance

As well as being an activist and propagandist, MacKinnon, like her father, was an accomplished lawyer. She understood how the law could be used as a powerful weapon to achieve political goals, regardless of whether the facts, or public sentiment, are on your side. MacKinnon and Dworkin opposed obscenity laws, which were based on moral judgements by trial juries. Obscenity laws based on a 'community standard' tend to weaken as public attitudes become more liberal; the pro-censorship feminists sought a way to attack sexual expression that didn't rely on public attitudes.

Instead, they opted to use (or, perhaps more accurately, abuse) civil-rights law. Since they argued that the very existence of pornography was harmful to women, they set out to create a law that would allow women claiming harm to sue for damages. They drafted a model law – the Antipornography Civil Rights Ordinance – that could be implemented by city and state governments.

The effects of such a law would be far more sweeping than obscenity laws. If a woman claimed to have had her civils rights violated in some way by pornography, she could punitively sue the studio, distributors and retailers. Whereas obscenity law attempts to set a community standard for what is acceptable, now a single individual could take action based on her own personal standards of decency.

As discussed earlier, it is difficult (if not impossible) to define the word pornography objectively, so the ordinance set out to create a definition. But its concept of porn was extremely broad, included not just imagery, but words, and provided eight, highly subjective, definitions of pornography, including:

"women are presented dehumanized as sexual objects, things or commodities" – which on its own could cover almost any form of erotica.

"women are presented as sexual objects experiencing sexual pleasure in rape, incest, or other sexual assault" – as we have seen, Dworkin considered all pornography to be sexual assault.

"women are presented in postures or positions of sexual submission, servility, or display" – again, this is subjective language, and could cover almost any erotic image, or even a clothed photograph of a woman that might be considered sexually submissive.

"women's body parts—including but not limited to vaginas, breasts, or buttocks—are exhibited such that women are reduced to those parts" – the phrase "but not limited to" means that a close-up image of a mouth, a shoulder, a knee, or an ankle could be considered pornographic.

"women are presented in scenarios of degradation, humiliation, injury, torture, shown as filthy or inferior, bleeding, bruised or hurt in a context that makes these conditions sexual" – contains a strange mix of specific scenarios (bleeding, bruised) with vague, catch-all terms (degradation, inferior).

It is hard to imagine any kind of expression related to sex or sexuality that could not be interpreted to fall within the Dworkin/MacKinnon definition of pornography. Museums displaying ancient Roman sculpture might be just as liable to being sued as adult video shops. Bookshops would have to bar work featuring any mention of sex at all, in case any sexual reference was deemed by anybody to be pornographic. Magazine covers featuring women in poses considered sexual – whether aimed at men or women – would have to be censored.

Furthermore, while modern obscenity laws make allowances for artistic expression, MacKinnon expressly ruled this out: "If a woman is subjected, why should it matter if the work has other value?"[19] So who could be sued under the law? It specified four broad targets:

First, anyone "trafficking" in porn – in other words, people selling, renting, publishing or exhibiting sexual material.

Second, anyone deemed to have coerced a woman into porn. If this seems reasonable at first glance, one should keep in mind that rape and kidnap were already illegal. The law would allow any model to later claim that they been coerced, even if they had signed consent forms and accepted payment, and to claim punitive damages. Since it would be in a model's financial interest to later claim coercion and sue, the end result of such a law would be to raise the risk and cost of making or selling porn to the point where it became effectively impossible.

Third, "forcing pornography on a person". Here, things get strange. Anyone who unintentionally sees any kind of sexual imagery could claim to have been damaged. Such a law would prevent any kind of public display of anything that anybody might deem to be sexual. In a recent story about "sexualisation of the high street" on the *Guardian* website, readers were asked to submit sexualised images. One reader submitted a photograph of a mannequin in a shop window with erect nipples. Under the ordinance, the shop would face a risk of being sued for damages.

Fourth, "assault or physical attack due to pornography". And here, things get stranger still. Although nobody had (or has still) provided an evidential link between pornography and violence, the claim of a link is often made. Sometimes, the link is even made by perpetrators of violence such as rapists or killers. This is hardly surprising: surely it is easier to blame somebody other than oneself when one has committed a horrible crime? Under this law, a rapist could blame his actions on having watched *Busty Sluts #7* the previous night. The producer of *Busty Sluts #7* could be sued and ruined. And the rapist? Logically, it was not his fault, so why should he be punished?

This might seem far-fetched, but in fact, anti-porn feminism inevitably leads to a position in which men are not to blame for their actions, reversing years of progressive efforts to ensure that rapists be held fully responsible for their crimes. MacKinnon actually argued that a particularly brutal individual, Thomas Schiro, who raped and killed a woman in 1981, should be found not-guilty, as he had watched porn and was therefore not responsible for his actions. She argued instead that the creators of the pornography that Schiro had watched were culpable.[20]

In a nutshell, the Antipornography Ordinance would effectively prevent anybody publishing any potentially sexual imagery, in case somebody found it 'degrading', 'humiliating', 'objectifying' or any of the other catch-all concepts it contained.

As a civil law rather than a criminal one, it would move censorship powers from the state into the hands of self-selected individuals. Any motivated person or group would be able to close down a sex shop or museum exhibition, prevent the publication of a book or likewise censor anything else they deemed to be pornographic. Anybody who dared to create, publish or disseminate sexual material would face financial destruction.

In 1983, the city of Minneapolis was the first to pass a law based on the Dworkin/MacKinnon model ordinance, but the mayor vetoed it. Further cities followed, and successfully implemented the law, but it was struck down each time under the First Amendment to the US Constitution.

In Praise of the First Amendment

United States history is short, endlessly bizarre and often brutal, but also full of surprises. The country is among the most conservative and religious in the Western World. Many religious Americans are uncomfortable with the existence of pornography; yet America is the hub of the global porn industry, and throughout its history the country has been the originator of some of the most revolutionary and subversive art, music and literature.

It appears to be a paradox: how can a nation be home to many of the world's most intolerant groups, ideas and people, and simultaneously be the strongest defender of free expression? The answer lies in the First Amendment to the Constitution, which simply states:

> Congress shall make no law respecting an establishment of religion, or prohibiting the free exercise thereof; or abridging the freedom of speech, or of the press; or the right of the people peaceably to assemble, and to petition the Government for a redress of grievances.

The First Amendment is frequently tested in the court system, and has been clarified by court decisions over time. Freedom of speech and of the press now extend to all forms of expression, including digital communications, and they now apply to individual state legislatures as well as the US Congress.

Not all expression is protected by the First Amendment: exceptions have crept in as a result of court decisions over the years. One such exception is 'obscenity', defined according to a community standard, much as in the United Kingdom. But pornography (other than that deemed to be obscene) is considered to be protected speech. In practise, this means that any outright attempt to ban pornography in the United States (such as that undertaken by Andrea Dworkin and Catharine

MacKinnon) is almost inevitably doomed to fail.

The First Amendment is not a simple line in the sand that protects freedom of expression in an unambiguous way – it is more accurately viewed as a battleground, on which the defence of free expression must be constantly fought. Yet, the very existence of this short paragraph of text has created space for minorities – including porn makers – to create and propagate material that the majority of the population may consider unacceptable or immoral.

The Antipornography Civil Rights Ordinance, despite being presented as a law to protect women, was a blatant attempt at censorship, thus breached the First Amendment and failed to take hold. America had been inoculated by its founding fathers against the virus of censorship. Not all countries are so lucky – least of all Britain, which is easily panicked, on a regular basis, into accepting ever-greater levels of censorship.

Gail Dines in Pornland

The MacDworkinites had been thwarted in their goal of censoring pornography in the United States, but the ideas they created have been spread internationally by a new generation of disciples. The best-known name in this area today is Gail Dines, a US-based author and academic of British origin. Dines has written two books on the subject of pornography, and regularly features on a variety of international media platforms.

Dines' 2010 book, *Pornland: How Porn Has Hijacked Our Sexuality* perhaps represents today's publication of choice for pro-censorship feminism; and there is certainly competition in this field. The porn-panic business appears to be a lucrative one.

I have met Dines twice in online debate; having heard so much about her, I was somewhat daunted to meet her, and thus very surprised to discover how little understanding she has of pornography or the porn industry, subjects she claims to have devoted over two decades of her academic life to studying.

Similarly, the British feminist porn director Anna Span debated against Dines at the University of Cambridge, and won the vote on a comfortable margin.

Pornland's overall thesis is that a huge, rich and powerful porn industry is deliberately manipulating and actually altering human sexuality in order to make a profit. This is some claim: re-engineering human sexuality and other aspects of inbuilt human behaviour could solve, or create, many problems for society. However, Dines provides no evidence to show that this has taken place. As an academic researching porn, Dines must be aware of the lack of evidence linking pornography to harm, but in *Pornland*, she hides this awareness with skill.

In order to demonstrate that the porn industry is immensely powerful (powerful enough to deliberately alter the human psyche, no less), Dines must present some impressive-looking financial figures; and she delivers, stating:

> The size of the porn industry is staggering. Though reliable numbers are hard to find, the global industry has been estimated to be worth around $96 billion in 2006, with the U.S. market worth approximately $13 billion... pornography revenues rival those of all the major Hollywood studios combined.[21]

These are impressive numbers indeed! And entirely fictional. The 'porn is bigger than Hollywood' myth is often quoted, and is a long way from the truth. In 2001, estimates were flying around of an industry worth between $10 to $14 billion, and these were dismissed by Forbes magazine[22] as a huge exaggeration. Forbes pointed out that the only reliable study, carried out in 1998 by Forrester, had estimated the industry size at between $750 million and $1 billion. The industry certainly grew impressively between 1998 and 2006; but a hundredfold? The fact that Dines could happily present such grossly incorrect figures is revealing of her agenda.

What is the quoted source of Dines' $96 billion number? A website[23] that reviews filtering software for parental control of Internet access. And what is *their* source? "Data based on a 2006 study." The name of the study is not provided, nor is a link to the study. So the key number underlying an entire anti-porn thesis is lifted from a website promoting porn filters which fails to even provide a source. And this is not just any book: *the* flagship book from *the* author who is the best-known anti-porn campaigner on the planet. Dines also fails to mention that the industry has been shrinking rapidly since about 2007, due to the rising availability of free pornography online.

The rest of *Pornland* possesses little more accuracy, but it is entertaining – comedic even. It features plenty of text apparently copied and pasted from adult websites. A sceptical reader could find contradictions and other logic problems on almost any page. The only thing that might prevent the reader from laughing out loud is that this book is being used to justify censorship of the Internet for entire countries, and its author boasts of providing advice to governments on the effects of pornography – a subject she appears not to know a huge amount about.

Other than vastly exaggerating the size and power of the porn industry, another core tenet of *Pornland* is that pornography is becoming more and more extreme. The only problem for Dines is that the reverse is true. In fact, as the industry has consolidated and come into the mainstream, many of the rough (and interesting) edges have been taken off it, to the detriment of many minority sexual fetishists, who have seen their own tastes attacked as obscene or extreme.

In making her various claims of harm, Dines ends up making contradictory points: on one hand, that content is becoming more extreme to feed a growing demand to see women brutalised; and on the other, that the industry is insidiously penetrating the mainstream by becoming less dirty.

How did this shift to the mainstream happen? The answer is simple: by design. What we see today is the result of years of careful strategizing by the porn industry by stripping away the "dirt" factor and reconstituting porn as fun, edgy, chic, sexy, and hot. The more sanitized the industry became, the more it seeped into the pop culture and into our collective consciousness.[24]

So we learn that porn is becoming more abusive and extreme, while simultaneously (and sneakily) selling itself as more fun, sanitised and mainstream. Dines fails to mention recent trends for feminist porn, ethical porn, porn for couples and 'romance porn'. Nor does she acknowledge that the industry is increasingly dominated by amateurs shooting and uploading their own content, rather than by larger production companies.

Her claim that the growth of the porn business is the result of 'careful strategizing' would amuse anyone who has had direct involvement with the industry. Just as in any entertainment industry, what is supplied is led by consumer demand. The industry is packed with producers trying to create new things, and hoping they will sell. Dines' near-religious view of humanity is that powerful and complex sexualities are not innate to us, but are instead planted in us by pornography (by which she means sexual expression in general). If the porn goes away, she appears to believe, so will our unhealthy, oppressive sexual fantasies and desires.

Despite repeatedly mentioning her two decades of study ("Although I have been studying the porn industry for over two decades... Through my experience lecturing on pornography for over two decades..."), Dines demonstrates some very basic misunderstandings of the industry and its terminology. The entire book is based around what she calls 'gonzo porn', which she writes "depicts hard-core, body-punishing sex in which women are demeaned and debased". But in fact, this is not what gonzo means at all. It actually refers to an impromptu, unscripted shooting style using hand-held cameras, often held by cast members themselves. The term references gonzo journalism, as practised by the likes of Hunter S. Thompson, in which the reporter is a part of the story he tells. This basic mistake in terminology again underlines Dines' lack of knowledge in her subject area, and even a lack of curiosity about it.

To confuse things even further, Dines makes assertions about 'gonzo porn' but then blurs the line between gonzo and all other pornography. To Dines, all pornography is bad, and when I met her in online debate[25], she stated that she wanted to see the entire porn industry destroyed, not just the parts controlled by big companies, or the parts that make rough porn. All of it.

Having made her claim that imagery is becoming more extreme, and thus more dangerous, she then claims that softer imagery is as dangerous as the more extreme variety:

[*Playboy* and *Penthouse*], with their soft-core, soft-focus pictures of naked women, taught boys and men that women existed to be looked at, objectified, used, and put away till next time.

Dines frequently reminds the reader that she is a feminist, and that she cares for the performers:

Some argue that assault is too strong a word, but if we analyze what is actually going on in a gonzo scene in a way that speaks to the experiences of the woman in the movie, then we get some insight into what is happening to her as a human being.

Yet Gail Dines shows little apparent interest in talking to these supposed victims of assault, or meeting any of the women or men who work in the porn industry, or attending a studio and seeing a shoot for herself. In her refusal to ask about their own, first-hand accounts of their experiences, she shows disdain for the women in the industry, while claiming to be their defender.

The closest Dines appears to have to come to the porn industry was to attend an industry convention in Las Vegas in January 2008. Her account of the show comes close to comic self-parody. She is clearly disgusted by everything she sees, and so (she tells us) is a middle-aged, African-American security guard called Patricia, who (we learn) agrees with everything Dines says about the porn industry. It appears not to have occurred to Dines that Patricia's expertise on pornography is perhaps even less than her own, or that she may have learned more by taking the chance to interview pornstars rather than security guards.

No matter. Patricia, we discover, is suffering a porn-related ailment: a "crick in her neck from trying to avoid looking at the porn that is being projected onto the screens". Further, we read that "Divorced for many years, Patricia tells me that after doing this job for a few days, she now knows why she 'can't find a good man to settle down with'".

Black female literature and magazines often focus on the alleged shortage of 'good men'. Now, thanks to Gail Dines (and Patricia), we know the root of the problem: porn has taken them all.

Pornland informs us that Patricia is now planning "her future far away from Las Vegas". My own black American friends are concerned with many things, including racism, low pay, lack of access to good healthcare, police harassment and the fear that their male relatives will be sent to prison, in common with one in three of all black American men. But (Dines tells us) Patricia, working a minimum-wage job in Las Vegas, is concerned about nothing more than porn, and may actually relocate to avoid it.

Censorship as a Weapon

Like Dworkin and Mackinnon before her, Dines believes in attacking her opponents' right to free speech. She believes not just in censoring porn, but also in censoring people who oppose her point of view.

Upon discovering that an adult-industry conference would be taking place in a London hotel in September 2013, she wrote to the hotel management claiming that their female employees would be put at risk by the very presence of pornographers in their hotel. She then posted the letter – another masterpiece in comic self-parody – to her Facebook campaign page[26]:

ACTION ALERT LETTER. Here is the letter I am sending. PLEASE re-send to custserv@radisson.com saying you are endorsing it.

Dear Radisson Board Members,

As a professor who studies the effects of pornography, and as a founding member of Stop Porn Culture (SPC), an international feminist anti-pornography organisation, I am writing on behalf of over 2,000 members to protest your hotel hosting the XBIZ porn conference in London on 22-25th September. We are outraged that you would provide space to an industry that is based on making a profit from brutalizing women. Moreover, pornography puts all women at risk by teaching men that women only have value as sexual objects, are always available as willing participants, and are thus legitimate targets of sexual harassment, abuse and rape. You are [especially] putting at risk all the female employees who work at your hotel during the XBIZ conference because men who sexually abuse women for profit will be staying at your hotel, eating in your hotel, and will be in close proximity to women employees who work at your hotel so they can feed themselves and their families. Please take this letter as a warning notice regarding these risks. Should a female employee be the victim of sexual harassment or assault, then your knowledge of these risks will increase your negligence and liability. SPC members will be writing to you endorsing this letter, as well as writing about this on vacation and other review websites urging potential customers to stay away from your hotels. Should you ignore this letter, our campaign could cause serious damage to your reputation and revenue. Please consider this before you provide a venue to an industry that does serious damage to the health and wellbeing of women and children.

Dines thus reveals her contempt for free speech. Not only can she not tolerate the dissemination of pornography, but she cannot even accept that people have the right to meet and *talk about* pornography. I have attended the London XBIZ conference, and it is a place in which men and women meet to discuss business, as well as politics, law and other industry-related issues. Ironically, the 2013 conference that Dines tried to disrupt was a forum for discussions about censorship, and was well attended by journalists as well as business people, lawyers and government regulators.

In passing, the use of the deeply unfeminist phrase "women and children" might be noted. The thin feminist veneer has slipped, revealing a deeply moralistic and patriarchal attitude towards 'the weaker sex'.

Slut-Shaming

Dines, in common with other anti-sex feminists, cannot decide whether pornstars are innocent victims to be saved, or slutty women who are to blame for men committing crimes of sexual and domestic violence. She engages in slut-shaming of which any religious fundamentalist would be proud, and in doing so reveals the conservative agenda that she tries so hard to hide beneath a superficially progressive message. Although she takes great pains in the preface to *Pornland* to deny that she is anti-sex, her dislike of sexuality clearly goes far further than simply its depiction in pornography.

In a multi-page account of *Girls Gone Wild*, an adult-entertainment label focusing on young, white 'frat girls' partying,

Dines writes:

> One of the major problems associated with being on *GGW* is that the young women's behaviour is forever frozen in time on tape; they can't take it back, hide it, or deny that they did it... the average female... gets treated not as a Paris Hilton wannabe but as a "slutty" girl who deserves to be ridiculed and shunned... One woman told me that after she had girl-on-girl sex with her friend, she felt like "a stupid whore and I can't stop people watching me. All the guys at school watch me and I feel horrible."[27]

Perhaps other feminists would be outraged by this sexist slut-shaming by the woman's college peers, but Dines has nothing to say about it. She does not blame the patriarchal, conservative-religious attitudes that are prevalent in American society. She does not defend the rights of the woman to have sex on camera if she chooses, without being stigmatised and attacked. Instead, she attacks the medium, and implicitly, the women themselves. After all, if they had not chosen to have sex on camera, nobody would now be branding them 'stupid whores'.

This attitude is repeated elsewhere in the book, and in Dines' other writings. One of the pieces of evidence she provides to show that porn has "seeped" into the public consciousness is that ex-pornstars have appeared in mainstream media:

> retired mega-porn star Jenna Jameson has written a best-selling book and appears in numerous popular celebrity magazines, and Sasha Grey, the new, more hard-core Jenna Jameson, is featured in a four-page article in *Rolling Stone* in May 2009 and appears in a Steven Soderburgh movie... Indiana University invites pornographer Joanna Angel to address a human sexuality class.

Dines disapproves of all of this: she apparently believes that, because these women have had sex on camera, they should be shunned by the media, universities and other respectable institutions. Once a slut, always a slut: hardly a message that most would recognise as a feminist one.

In 2011, the Slutwalk movement began in Toronto, in response to a police spokesperson who had commented: "women should avoid dressing like sluts in order not to be victimised". Within weeks, the movement had spread globally, and Slutwalk marches were being held in many cities. The message was simple: women have the right to choose to be sluts, without stigma, judgement or attack. If 'slut' simply refers to women who enjoy sex, then the word should be reclaimed from those who use it as a slur.

Slutwalk would act as a litmus test for feminists, splitting opinion along anti-sex/sex-positive lines. The marches featured women dressed in revealing, raunchy clothing, as well as their male supporters. Although its message was a feminist one – a woman's right to present and use her own body as she chooses – it also posed a challenge to anti-sex feminists, who believe that expressions of sexuality are themselves demeaning to women. How would Dines respond?

In a 2011 *Guardian* article[28], titled "Slutwalk is not sexual liberation", Gail Dines and Wendy J. Murphy dismissed Slutwalk and its goal of reclaiming 'sluttishness' from sexist and patriarchal attitudes. It is a masterpiece of buttoned-up-conservatism-as-feminism.

The piece begins: 'It wasn't long ago that being called a "slut" meant social death', before going on to make clear that it should remain that way:

> The organisers claim that celebrating the word "slut", and promoting sluttishness in general, will help women achieve full autonomy over their sexuality. But the focus on

"reclaiming" the word slut fails to address the real issue. The term slut is so deeply rooted in the patriarchal "madonna/whore" view of women's sexuality that it is beyond redemption.

But the pair are not just worried about the word – they make clear that they consider sluttish behaviour itself to be a betrayal:

The recent TubeCrush phenomenon, where young women take pictures of men they find attractive on the London tube and post them to a website, illustrates how easily women copy dominant societal norms of sexual objectification rather than exploring something new and creativeAnd [sic] it's telling that while these pictures are themselves innocent and largely free of sexual innuendo, one can only imagine the sexually aggressive language that would accompany a site dedicated to secret photos of women.

In other words, women cannot choose to be sexually liberated: any attempt to become so is merely an imitation of male sexual behaviour, and is thus not liberation. Sexual admiration of women by men is abusive, and women must take care to avoid following this bad example. The article dismisses both 'slut' and 'frigid' labels of female sexuality. How are women supposed to behave? Which expressions of female sexuality are acceptable? This is left unclear: the unwritten message is that all expression of sexuality is to be shunned, and pride in sluttishness is wrong: "Women need to take to the streets – but not for the right to be called 'slut'".

Via activists like Gail Dines, the message that sexual expression is harmful to women has taken root, and is undermining support for sexual freedom and free speech on the political left as well as on the right. Nowhere is this truer than in Britain.

The New British Anti-Sex Movement

Likewise also that women should adorn themselves in respectable apparel, with modesty and self-control – Timothy 2:9

Mary Whitehouse, the Christian morality campaigner, must have been dismayed by the increasingly liberal (or "permissive", to use her word of choice) attitudes that became prevalent in the 1990s. Although she had been influential in introducing video censorship in the 1980s, by the time she died in 2001, Britain had become a very different place. The Internet was delivering uncensored pornography (and every other form of content) into people's homes, bypassing state censorship efforts. Homosexuality had finally ceased to be treated as taboo: the singer George Michael was one of many celebrities who were outed or came out during the 1990s, without the damage to their career that would have resulted in any previous era. Religious belief was in steep decline, with 15% declaring themselves to be atheists in the 2001 census, but with a far larger proportion of society not following any religion in practice.

The arrival of the new Labour government in 1997 marked the start of a new British era. Conservatives had been in power since Thatcher's election victory in 1979. Now, Tony Blair, the young, charismatic new Prime Minister, signalled a political, social and generational shift. Britain suddenly seemed younger, more progressive, more urban: Cool Britannia had arrived, and the stuffy old homophobes and racists who had run the country for 18 years suddenly seemed to represent the past.

The *Daily Mail* continued to speak for the most conservative parts of middle England, but in the new Britain, the *Mail* seemed as old and irrelevant as the Conservative Party, and it was mocked rather than feared. We, a new, multiracial, tolerant generation, felt as if the country was ours for the first time, and it was a wonderful feeling. As in the 1960s, social conservatives seemed to be in retreat, once again being swept away by the tide of history. And as in the 1960s, social conservatives had little option but to watch the country change, to regroup, reinvent themselves, and bide their time.

Now that Britain had become a more progressive and secular society, conservatives needed a new message and new language in order to attack the sexual permissiveness that they saw around them. The battles over casual sex, contraception, abortion and homosexuality were all but over. The front-line for sexual freedom had now rolled into new territories, and in order to fight successfully, anti-sex conservatives had to capture support on the left as well as the right. *Daily Mail* readers needed no more convincing that 'permissiveness' was a problem, but how to win over *Guardian* readers?

Andrea Dworkin and Catharine MacKinnon had already laid the groundwork for a 'progressive' attack on sexual freedoms; now their messages and methods could be adopted and adapted for the UK.

A Tale of Two Feminists

The pornography debate panel in which I participated at UCL featured two feminists. Sitting next to me was the model, ex-pornstar and feminist, Renée Richards. On the other side of the panel was Julia Long from Object, a British anti-sex feminist group that attacks sexual expression in all its forms.

Richards described her years in the porn industry, and explained what it had been like to have sex on camera for a living. She outlined a typical day on set, from the bacon sandwiches and make-up sessions to the sex, explaining that each model sets his or her own 'levels' in advance: some performers will only work solo, or on girl–girl shoots. Others will work boy–girl, although some will only work with their own off-screen partner. Some will have anal sex, many won't. These levels are respected: any director who asks models to go beyond their levels will not be taken seriously in the industry for long. The industry is small, and the social networks are tight; anyone who is difficult or unpleasant to work with will quickly be notorious throughout the UK business.

Is the job dangerous? Richards suggested the opposite. One of the benefits of making porn, she said, was that she could test her sexual fantasies and limits in a safe environment. Many women fantasise about taking part in a 'gang bang'. Richards described how she was able to participate in a scene with five men and fulfil this fantasy, knowing that the performers and the crew would not push her further than she wanted to go, and that she could call a halt to the action at any time. In which other setting could such a fantasy be explored so safely?

What was the effect of porn-making on her self-esteem? Had she been reduced to a mere object, and had her confidence suffered as a result, as is so often suggested by anti-porn activists? Again, the opposite: Richards described her transformation from a shy teenager who would keep a T-shirt on during sex with her first boyfriend to an extrovert who loved to spend time naked. The not-quite-flat stomach that she had once tried to hide away was no longer a source of embarrassment to her.

Was there pressure to stay in the industry? In one way, yes: she outlined how she had had to make the adjustment from high earner to poor student when she decided to quit the industry. But quit she did, when she felt the time was right.

I was interested to hear Julia Long's perspective; how would she counter Richards' first-hand account? Ultimately, she did not try to. Nor did she have a response to my summary of statistics and research on pornography. Instead she gave a speech decrying the evils of the porn industry, in terms that seemed to have been inspired by MacKinnon, Dworkin and Dines; surprisingly, she seemed to have no direct knowledge of the industry at all. Her lack of understanding of the subject area contrasted sharply with Richards' first-hand account.

Long summed up by invoking an unnamed woman she had met, who had been a porn performer, and had been damaged by her experiences in unspecified ways. This use of anecdotes about nameless victims, I was to discover, is an old strategy that had been frequently employed in the past by Mary Whitehouse. I was surprised at how one-sided the debate had been, and so, it seemed, were the students in attendance. Renée and I easily won the debate on a show of hands.

I had heard much about Object previously, and I wanted to make contact with them and try to arrange a meeting to exchange views and ideas. I felt that their misunderstandings of porn (and other sex entertainment industries) could perhaps be overcome by challenging their ignorance of the subject, and perhaps by introducing them to women working in the industry. When the meeting closed, I walked over to Long and her small group of supporters to introduce myself, but they glared at me and swept out of the hall before I could reach them.

This had been my second personal encounter with Object, the first having taken place a few months earlier. I had been attending an industry conference in central London, when shouting was heard outside, so I and a few others went to investigate. Object were holding a protest against Internet pornography; strangely, the protesters were shouting about rapes in the Democratic Republic of Congo, a war-torn country that has experienced a tsunami of war-related sexual violence against women, children and men. I say strangely, because DRC has among the lowest Internet usage of any country. In fact, electricity is relatively rare, and much of the country cannot even be reached by road. In other words, DRC must have among the lowest levels of access to pornography in the world, so it was bizarre to link Internet pornography with its truly horrific rape epidemic.

I was joined on the pavement by Liselle Bailey, one of Britain's best-known female porn directors, and we approached the woman who was apparently leading the protest. "Would you like to talk to a female porn director?" I asked.

The woman screamed something about rape at me, then turned her back. I approached a couple of others, with similar results. Only one woman was prepared to talk to me. Unlike the others, who seemed uniformly white and middle-class, she was dark-skinned, and had a cockney accent. She explained that her mother had been a sex worker, and she hated the sex trade. We chatted for a little while, and she remarked that I seemed like a person with a good heart, in response to which I offered to hug her. She lifted her arms towards me, then rapidly dropped them again. "I'd better not", she said, indicating the shouting protesters around her, some of whom were glaring in our direction. And she turned away.

Object and UK Feminista

Early in the new century, not long after Mary Whitehouse had died, a private party was underway at Browns, a well-known East London strip venue. To the astonishment of the party-goers, a small but noisy protest began outside. The protest was led by Anna van Heeswijk, who later went on to set up Object. The party was being held to celebrate the birthday of the bar manager, a gay man, and the only strippers were male. Stripper and activist Edie Lamort recalls:

> The dancers started laughing at them and told them they had come on the wrong night, 'Hahaha there are male strippers here if you want to check them out!' But the haters kept on shouting outside, on a cold November night.

Object was dismissed by the dancers as a small, unrepresentative group of morality campaigners, which was, and still is, an

77

accurate assessment. But political power is far more about connections and finance than the strength of grassroots support, and the anti-strip-club activists began to gain influential supporters. Harriet Harman, a senior figure in the Labour government, was a supporter of sexual-morality causes, including calls for the criminalisation of the sex trade, and she helped push through a change to licensing law that would make it harder to acquire a license for a strip club. The legal change inspired the morality campaigners, and they began to push for councils in the East London boroughs of Hackney and Tower Hamlets to withdraw licenses from existing clubs.

As with the 1980s MacDworkinite anti-porn campaigns in America, the new groups – including Object and UK Feminista – packaged their campaign as a women's-rights one, to win over liberal support and deflect from accusations that they were continuing the morality work of the religious right. And as the MacDworkinites had done, they shared platforms with religious conservatives. Edie Lamort recalls attending public meetings aimed at closing down the strip venues:

> these people are trying to take us back 100 years or so. And they sit up there on panels, next to religious fundamentalists and I think: What are you doing? Can't you see you'll be next? If you succeed in your mission to ban all of us and persecute all of us, it will close in around you as well. You are only free because we are free!

Object and UK Feminista drew on the tactics that MacKinnon and Dworkin had developed in their earlier struggles. They painted the striptease industry as an oppressive male-run business in which women are exploited and abused; yet it was hard to make this stand up, as many of London's strip venues, including Browns, the location of Object's first protest, were owned and run by women.

The prohibitionists also failed to produce victims who would help them demonstrate the exploitative nature of the striptease industry. Indeed, the response of the East London strippers to the campaign was to join trade unions and fight to defend their workplaces and their jobs.

In response to this, the feminist campaigners became increasingly hostile towards the dancers – odd behaviour indeed from people calling themselves women's-rights activists. They alleged that the dancers were in the pay of their 'pimps', and that they had been so abused and controlled that they had developed Stockholm Syndrome – a psychological condition in which a kidnap victim develops positive feelings towards her kidnapper. In other words, they clearly believed that the views of the women who worked in the strip venues were not worth listening to, and they did their best to silence and suppress the strippers' voices.

This refusal to listen to the women that they claim to be saving is a common factor in the campaigning of Object and UK Feminista, as well as in their supportive media. The groups are remarkably dismissive towards women who disagree with their views. I asked Edie Lamort about the prohibitionists' failure to ask how the dancers themselves felt.

Nobody ever asks us... it's one of the things we find most offensive about Object and UK Feminista. And when we do try to talk to them and try to say 'hold on a second, this is our point of view', they accuse us of having Stockholm Syndrome. The debate I went to [in Tower Hamlets]... they told me I was a propagandist for the sex industry and my pimp must have paid me to do it. I said, 'No, nobody's paying me! I'm doing this for free. I wish somebody would pay me!'

Another stripper and trade-unionist, Shelley, told me:

It does seem very wrong that they're trying to dictate what we can do to earn a living, what we can do with our bodies, how we can express ourselves and making such extreme judgements on what we can do. Basically telling us that we don't have the right to choose what we're doing. And I think that the biggest insult that we've heard against us is the idea that any dancer who says she enjoys what she does is the ultimate example of just how abused we are, without even realising it, how we're suffering from Stockholm Syndrome, we're in love with our abusers... it's just massively insulting!

Shelley became an activist in the campaign to save the strip clubs, and attended a consultation in Parliament, where she encountered anti-sex feminists:

I'd gone with a friend. After we left the meeting we didn't even speak to each other... we were just so horrified by what we'd heard. We as dancers had been talked about in such a derogatory manner by Object. It felt like being punched in the stomach. We had been labelled as being victims, and on the other hand, evil women who were the cause of rape and abuse... It feels like emotional abuse. I've never felt like an object in a derogatory sense; my audiences certainly never made me feel like that. The only people who have labelled me in that way, and made me feel like that, are Object and similar feminist groups.

Shelley recalled with anger that the prohibitionists she encountered had never even stepped inside a strip club.

To have another woman who actually hasn't been in a strip club, who won't hear my voice, won't hear my side of it, because what I'm saying is just proof of how 'abused' I am... to have someone like that telling me that what I've been doing for the last 10 years is the root cause of virtually all the ills in society... 'You're the cause of rape, you're the cause of abuse, you're the cause of domestic violence! It's all because of what *you've* been doing!'

In order to back the claim that strip clubs caused harm, prohibitionists drew heavily on the 'Lilith Report', a 2003 study by Lilith R&D/Eaves, which suggested a link between the existence of strip clubs in an area and the prevalence of rape. The report was quickly seized on by morality campaigners to show that sexual expression was harmful to women. But the report was deeply flawed, and included data only from years that showed increases in rape while ignoring years that showed decreases. It was torn apart by the sex writer and researcher Dr Brooke Magnanti, who looked at the same data and found a fall, rather than a rise, in rape when correlated against strip clubs opening. Yet Magnanti is a scientist, and was honest enough to point out that a correlation is not a causation; in other words, her findings did not prove that strip clubs reduce rapes; but they certainly showed that they were not linked to an increase. The Lilith Report was thoroughly discredited, and yet continued and still continues to be used by prohibitionists. Ten years later, Object still referenced it on their website.[29]

How Sex Panics Are Created

A tour of the Object website[30] was a lesson in the power of sensational claim over rational argument. The site was packed with claims and insinuations of harm for which no evidence is provided. Object was masterful at hinting about links between sexual expression and various societal problems (or perceived problems) without actually justifying the links made.

A page headed "The Facts" provided a wonderful lesson in propaganda. After I wrote a blog post about the contents of the page, most of the "facts" I commented on were removed. The original page contained a list of facts without any explanation as to how these relate to Object's campaigns. For example:

Over half (54%) of all women around the world say they first became aware of the need to be physically attractive between 6 and 17 years of age.

This is characteristic of the confusing way in which anti-sex propaganda is presented by groups like Object. Firstly, note the wide age range. Young children are deliberately grouped together with young adults in order to give the impression that children are being 'sexualised'. Such a wide age range is effectively meaningless in such a context: worse, it is troubling that attitudes of prepubescent children are being grouped with those of legal adults. Second – and this is incredibly common in propaganda designed to generate moral panic – no trends are given. In order to demonstrate a change for the worse, the numbers must be compared with past values. Does 54% represent a fall or rise in this metric? No clue is given, although almost everything Object says is designed to panic people, to create the impression that things are getting worse. Is 54% a high number? Most people learn about the importance of building social status during their childhood and teenage years. And like it or not, part of what determines one's social status – regardless of gender – is attractiveness. This may not be fair, or nice, but it is human behaviour. It is likely that such instincts are in part the result of evolution, rather than porn, or lap dancing, or 'sexualised' advertising, or any of the other things that Object opposes. But there is no interpretation provided of what this 'fact' means. They just state it, as if it somehow makes their case. Let's try another:

Eating disorders are as common among women as autism.

What does this tell us about eating disorders? Or about autism?

From the little I have read on both subjects, it seems that both types of disorder are often genetic in origin, and autism is more prevalent in men than in women. So what are Object trying to say here? I have no idea.

66% of teenage girls would consider plastic surgery and 20% would do it right now.

Is this a lot? Is this number rising or falling, and why?

Polls suggest that 63% of young women aspire to be glamour models or lap dancers.

That sounds high. But we know that poll results depend on the question asked. After I blogged about this point, I was contacted by Dr Petra Boynton, a social psychologist who specialises in sex and relationships, who told me the figure was false, having been lifted from a 2005 poll created to promote a mobile entertainment company. She had blogged[31] about the poll, highlighting its inaccuracy. Young women had actually been asked whether they would rather be Abi Titmuss (a young model and actress), Germaine Greer (a feminist author and academic in her 60s) or Anita Roddick (a businesswoman also in her 60s). Of course, most young women would identify more with somebody around their own age. It was meaningless fluff designed to generate press coverage, but from Object's point of view, it constituted evidence.

Try as I might, I couldn't find any firm evidence on the site to back any of the claims Object were making about the harmfulness of sexual expression. I've read a good number of articles by members of Object and UK Feminista, by Gail Dines, and other anti-sex activists, and the pattern remains the same: endless sensational claims of harm but no evidence provided to support them.

Searching For Victims

Morality campaigners have searched for decades for the smoking gun: that piece of research that demonstrates sexual images and videos can be harmful. They have failed to find it, and their approaches to campaigning are an open admission of that fact. Advocates of censorship, especially in the more religious United States, continuously accuse one medium after another of corrupting its consumers.

Erotic literature, rock and roll, hip hop, computer games, horror films, heavy metal, dance music, violent films and many other art-forms have all been accused of undermining societal values and causing bad behaviour. In 2013, the evangelical American Pastor John Hagee was still warning his congregations that *Harry Potter* books are "opening the gates of your mind to the Prince of Darkness and he will invade, and once he's invited in, he doesn't go out until he is cast out".[32] Hagee also warned in the same sermon that rock-and-roll music was "Satanic cyanide", which suggested he might be a little out of touch with popular culture.

Authoritarians continually prod at the public consciousness, looking for ways to ignite a panic that can be used to justify censorship. Object, UK Feminista and their sister groups around the world represent the latest round in that endless battle. In a rational society, claims of harm are not instantly swallowed with no evidence to back them.

Their first port of call in the search for evidence of harm was to find performers who had been genuinely harmed by the sex industries. As we have seen, Linda Marchiano was adopted by Dworkin and MacKinnon to attack the porn industry, even though her abuser was her husband, who was not a pornographer. Since Marchiano, the anti-porn lobby has failed to find many high-profile victims, other than the nameless ones that they cite during public meetings and parliamentary enquiries.

This raises a question: if Object and similar groups genuinely have evidence of abuse taking place on porn sets and in strip clubs, why do they not report it to the authorities? Why have there been no arrests of strip-club owners or porn producers? It is a virtual certainty that such a story would be splashed across newspaper front pages, and triumphantly promoted by the pro-censorship lobby. It is surely a tenet of feminism that rapists and sexual abusers should face justice, so why do *these* feminists not help bring *these* abusers to trial? Are they covering for sexual abuse? Or else, fabricating it?

In October 2014, I published an open letter[33] to the CEO of Object to address the issue of their use of rape allegations:

> This is an open letter to Roz Hardie, CEO of the campaign group Object.
> Dear Roz,
> ...I'm contacting you to suggest an alliance in one area where we seem to agree, and where we can work together against one of the great scourges of society: rape.
> You see, in all the years I've been following Object, I've noticed your frequent claims that women in the sex enter-tainment industries are being raped as a matter of routine...
> Object seem to have one core tactic: to shout "rape" in the context of pornography and other sexual entertainment...
> At your protest last Saturday, your supporters were screaming "rapist" at men walking into [the strip club] Spearmint Rhino. There were also women going into the club, and curiously your people called them "losers". I would have expected that, if you believed women were being raped in Spearmint Rhino, you would be extending an arm of support to them, rather than screaming childish insults.
> It has long troubled me that Object are prepared to make endless claims of rape and sexual abuse against the sex enter-tainment industries; and yet, to my knowledge, you have filed no police reports. Nobody has been arrested or taken to court.

Shouldn't rapists face the full might of the law? As we know, rape convictions are difficult to get, because it often comes down to one person's word against another. But you're claiming that industrial-scale rape is taking place ON VIDEO! Surely, convictions will be easy in these cases?

So here's my proposal: if, as you have long claimed, Object have evidence of sexual violence associated with the sexual entertainment industries, then let's approach the police with it. I will help you identify the publishers, producers and performers involved. We recently discovered that we both live in the same London borough – shall we fix a date to meet at [our local] police station?

As a "feminist human rights organisation", I've no doubt you will leap at the chance of bringing rapists to the attention of the law. If, on the other hand, you are merely using rape accusations as a tool of panic in order to further moralistic, pro-censorship aims, then you are taking the fight against sexual violence backward rather than forward. By labelling random men as rapists, and by referring to consenting sex between adults as rape, you are redefining the concepts of rape and consent to suit a conservative, anti-sex agenda. By harassing women who work in the sex industries, while telling the media that you are "saving" them, you divert attention away from sexual violence and towards the stigma-tisation of healthy, adult sexual expression.

A female business owner who witnessed your behaviour on Saturday wrote the following to me:

"Object's attitude towards anyone, whether they are remotely affiliated to the adult industry or directly involved in it, is absolutely disgusting. A couple of guys were horrified when they arrived as they had the term 'Rapist' shouted at them. It is irresponsible to use such terms so candidly when a number of women and some men even have been subjected to such horrible crime. It is dangerous and potentially damaging to society when people start using such labels so lightly. Most will agree that this is not a rational way of putting across any sort of argument, this is quite simply verbal abuse because our ideals of sexual freedom and freedom of speech are not line with theirs."

I look forward to hearing from you, and helping you ensure that the violent criminals you regularly invoke are brought to justice...

Although Object tweeted me, promising a response in due course, none was received.

Certainly, there are individuals who regret their earlier work in pornography or striptease. In an industry that has employed (at least) hundreds of thousands of people in the past few decades, that is hardly surprising.

It can also be noted that there is good money to be earned in 'victim porn'. Newspapers that refuse to write sympathetically about sex workers, pornstars and strippers are often more than happy to host columns written by women who have horror stories to tell. Shelley (herself an ex-journalist) notes that the media and morality campaigners have no interest in hearing the voices of strippers:

unless you're saying 'I hate it all and it was terrible and it was traumatic', in which case they'll listen to you and say, 'Oh poor you' – any other thing they just don't want to know about.

Despite the endless horror stories emanating from the anti-sex movement, real victims of the industry have been hard to find. Without hard evidence that the porn industry harms its female performers (and with the presence of plenty of performers who are prepared to defend their choice of career), prohibitionists have instead set out to broaden the meaning of the word 'harm', and demonstrate that pornography is somehow damaging to all women everywhere, not just those that work in front of the camera.

Redefining 'Harm'

At the foundation of any good moral panic must lie claims of harm. The mass media, an essential agent in creating panics, requires a simple story, or set of stories, in order to create the essential preconditions for the final Something-Must-Be-Done moment. The early attempts by the anti-porn movement to whip up outrage rested on the alleged harm done to performers. The failure of this strategy required new victims to be found, and the morality movement has been highly creative in finding them.

The first step was to misrepresent pornography as something created by men for men. This is doubly inaccurate: women have long been involved in the creation of sexual expression, and not just in front of the camera. Indeed, the baring of 'dangerous' female flesh has often been an element of feminist protest. There are increasing numbers of high-profile female, and feminist, porn directors, and even an increasingly popular Feminist Porn Awards ceremony and convention that runs annually in Toronto. Anti-porn feminists, especially Gail Dines, simply ignore the existence of these women: to acknowledge them would be to lose their simple 'men exploiting women' message. Similarly, gay porn is ignored; its existence is awkward for a movement based on the idea that porn is misogynistic.

On the consumption side, rising numbers of women enjoy pornography, and women are ever-more open to admitting and discussing their enjoyment of it. A *Marie Claire* study[34] published in October 2015 revealed that the vast majority of women surveyed (who were mostly under 34) viewed porn, with over 40% watching at least once a week.

Having misrepresented porn as an exclusively male interest, the pro-censorship movement must then create a link between the availability of pornography and harm done to women: they need to convince people that men who look at porn are more inclined to do harm to women. As will be seen, there is a lack of evidence to back this claim, but lack of evidence has never stood in the way of fundamentalists of any stripe. Instead, campaigners have made clever use of language to confuse the debate. A number of porn-panic keywords have come into being, or existing words repurposed, and by endless repetition in the media, have been pushed into the public consciousness.

Objectification

Among the most powerful of the porn-panic keywords is 'objectification'. *Wiktionary.org* defines *objectify* as follows:

1. to make something (such as an abstract idea) possible to be perceived by the senses
2. to treat as something objectively real
3. to treat as a mere object and deny the dignity of

The third definition is closest to the one people will think of in this context. A person who sees another as an object rather than a fellow human being may be more capable of committing harm against them. Thus the removal of somebody's humanity could well be harmful. It is likely that objectification plays some role in most violence, including sexual violence.

Objectification was first seized on by Dworkin and MacKinnon as a tool in their battle against sexual expression. They created the concept of sexual objectification, claiming that watching porn caused men to see women *in general* – not just those performing – as sex objects, which was harmful to all women. This idea assumes that men are not capable of distinguishing between women in pornography and other women they may encounter in their day-to-day lives. The idea was not backed by research, but it was a powerful propaganda tool, because it was easy to understand, and had the scope to generate fear without the need to provide evidence of harm. Objectification features prominently in today's moral panics over sexual expression.

As I have often discovered during discussions and debates, people who use the term tend to be certain that the sexual objectification is real, but oddly incapable of explaining how it works in practise.

Clarissa Smith is Professor of Sexual Cultures at Sunderland University, and has run (along with two other British academics) the biggest study into the effects of pornography on its users ever undertaken in Britain. When I asked her about the anti-porn version of objectification – that men look at sexual imagery and then are more likely to regard women as objects merely for sexual pleasure – her reply was straightforward: "That would be to assume men are beyond autistic". Indeed, the fundamental thinking behind this version of objectification is to label men as both stupid and dangerous. Many men, rather than reject this stereotyping, instead buy into the myth and respond with guilt: "I enjoy porn, and it hasn't turned me into a rapist, but if it does so to other men, then perhaps something should be done about it".

Shelley has often thought about this question during her years working as a stripper:

> I went to an all-girls school. I was made to believe that most men were terrible, all after one thing. And my opinion of men has actually gone *up* through being involved in this industry. I think they're fantastic. And I'm outraged on their behalf that they're all being labelled in such a negative way.

What should arouse suspicion is that objectification only seems to apply in sexual contexts. I have never heard complaints that women are objectified when they appear as ballet dancers or sprinters, for example. In this way of thinking, men are capable of seeing women's athletics without assuming all women are athletes, but are incapable of seeing some women presented sexually without assuming all women are objects for nothing other than sexual pleasure.

The close links between anti-sex feminism and religious morality have become apparent as Christian morality campaigners increasingly abandon their old warnings of eternal hellfire, and instead appropriate feminist language. Now, instead of warning youngsters that they would go to hell for dressing immodestly, they seize on objectification instead. A 2013 article in *Christianity Today* for example, titled "A Dad's Perspective: Why I Tell My Daughters to Dress Modestly", includes the following:

> Our bodies are not sinful or problematic—they are created by God and are beautiful things. Still, for many people, the bodies of others are tempting and cause them to think about that person in an objectified, sexualized light.[35]

Take away the bit about God, and this could appear on Object's website.

The misused concept of objectification – painting men as lustful brutes who are turned into rapists by the sight of the female form – represents the subversion of an existing idea. Other porn-panic words apparently are used only to create fear, and dispense with any meaningful definition. They mean whatever the user wants them to mean, which makes them powerful propaganda tools. The most popular of these words is sexualisation.

Sexualisation

For the past few years, it has become increasingly common to hear that 'sexualisation' is afflicting some aspect of our society.

The word is thrown around by pro-censorship campaigners and journalists in a wide variety of contexts. The most common early usage was the 'sexualisation of children', but as it has become more popular, the contexts for its use have multiplied. Now, our media, our high streets and our entire culture have – we are told – become sexualised.

The term is perfect for creating a moral panic: it is vague yet ominous. It has invaded and infected a wide range of discussions, from how children are dressed to the way magazines are sold in supermarkets. For anyone trying to understand what it actually means, it is infuriatingly difficult to pin down. In many minds, it is accepted as a simple fact that society/children/media have been sexualised. As one would expect from a well-formed moral panic, its advocates provide no solid evidence of the phenomenon's existence or its effects, and the mass media report it as fact, without any apparent curiosity as to why no evidence has been presented.

The term's popularity in the UK descends largely from a government study undertaken by Reg Bailey, and released in 2011 as the Bailey Review of the Commercialisation and Sexualisation of Childhood. The review made a series of recommendations related to restrictions on "sexualised imagery", including restrictions on the broadcast of "sexually explicit" music videos, censorship of magazine covers and further restrictions on TV content that is broadcast before the 9pm watershed.

The report's findings are often used by pro-censorship advocates as evidence that Something Bad is happening to our children and our society. For many commentators, the existence of the Bailey Review is demonstration enough that sexualisation is real and problematic, and that Something Must Be Done in response. However, Reg Bailey is the Chief Executive, not of a scientific research institution, but of Mothers' Union, which describes itself on its website as follows:

Mothers' Union is an international Christian charity that seeks to support families worldwide... For all 4 million members what Mothers' Union provides is a network through which they can serve Christ in their own community – through prayer, financial support and actively working at the grassroots level in programmes that meet local needs.

Readers may wonder why the UK government chose to appoint the head of a Christian campaigning organisation to determine whether children are being sexualised.

Does the Bailey Review have any scientific basis, or provide evidence to back up its calls for clampdowns on media? In a word, no – it is based on surveys of parental attitudes, not on scientific research either into media or into its effects on children. Certainly, parents' views are important, but such a report is hardly an authoritative study on social changes or their effects on children – and yet, it is used as one by commentators. Post-Bailey, sexualisation is widely accepted as fact, and has become the keyword of a widespread, growing moral panic over sexuality and sexual expression.

In her book *The Sex Myth*, sex researcher and author Dr Brooke Magnanti examined the Bailey Review, and concluded that:

It does not summarise any academic evidence regarding sexualisation...

It does not conduct new evidence seeking regarding the effects of early commercialisation or sexualisation...

It does offer the results of questionnaires and focus groups...

It does make a number of recommendations, purportedly based on the results of the questionnaires and focus groups;

however, close examination shows that in many cases, the responses do not support the changes suggested.[36]

The sexualisation claims are worth examining. One of the uses of the word is in the context of children wearing 'sexually provocative' clothing or makeup. But this seems to miss an important point. Lipstick or a mini-skirt on a child are not sexually provocative exactly because they are on a child. A skirt that might be sexy on a grown woman is sexy *because* it is on a grown woman.

It seems that a prepubescent child in a mini-skirt can only be sexual to a person with an unhealthy view of sexuality, and this apparently includes those people who refer to children wearing mini-skirts as 'sexualisation'. This is reinforced by the fact that, usually, only girls are deemed to be the victims of sexualisation. As a child, I spent the summers running around wearing little other than shorts, as many boys do today. Yet these boys are not held up as victims of sexualisation, while a girl of the same age, wearing a skirt and a vest, for example, might be. The very people sexualising young girls are those claiming to be trying to prevent it.

Similarly, sexualisation advocates have claimed to be upset that Playboy, an adult entertainment brand, has produced merchandise for children that features the famous Playboy bunny logo. But the bunny is not inherently sexual. It seems unlikely that Playboy writing paper acts as some kind of gateway device to lure children into a life of sleaze. Again, the only dodgy association seems to be in the minds of those who claim to have the children's interests at heart.

The old patriarchal message that says displays of the female body are in some way wrong has been carefully repackaged and sold as child protection. Having lost the old morality arguments that tried to shame women into wearing modest clothing, a new front has opened up, aimed at persuading children – or more specifically, girls – that their bodies are shameful, and must be hidden from sight. This is an old message indeed: only the language has been updated.

The attack on 'sexualised' music videos is based on similar thinking. In her videos, Beyoncé wears skimpy clothing and dances in a sexually provocative way. Dance is, after all, an inherently sexy art-form – and children have always learned to dance (and do most other things) by copying adults. This does not mean that a child who copies Beyoncé's dance moves is advertising herself as sexually available. She is doing what children do: copying adults in preparation for adulthood. In the official view, a video that shows an adult booty-shaking should not be seen by children because they too will booty-shake. And that, we are told (disturbingly), is a child being 'sexualised'.

Another version of sexualisation is (we are told) infecting the British high street. We are, according to increasingly frequent newspaper reports, being 'bombarded' with sexual imagery in public places, where we cannot avoid it. Although I have often looked out for this sexualisation, I have yet to find it. But still, the reports persist. The *Guardian*, generally seen as a liberal newspaper, has been responsible for some of the most dishonest articles behind the sexualisation panic. This reporting culminated in June 2013 with a crowd-sourcing exercise that was introduced in a style more often associated with the right-wing *Daily Mail*:

Are you offended by pornographic images on magazine and newspaper shelves in supermarkets and service stations? Have you spotted sexualised imagery you consider offensive on T-shirts or other goods on the high street? Does it make you angry that you and perhaps your kids too are inadvertently exposed to this kind of material by retailers as they go out and about?

The *Guardian* would like you to help document the story by looking for specific examples that you come across. If you care about the issue and would like to get involved, help us report the story by sharing photos of any problematic imagery you've seen in public.[37]

Would this exercise finally produce the evidence to back countless media stories about sexualisation? The images were published[38] a few days later and would have proved disappointing to anyone looking for proof that Britain's high streets had become sexualised. They consisted of multiple photographs of the *Daily Sport* and *Daily Star* tabloid newspapers, complete with bikini models on their covers; photographs of lads' mags, again with bikini shots; photographs of porn magazines; photographs of some billboards and T-shirts showing clothed models; more photographs of the *Sport*; more photographs of porn mags; more photographs of lads' mags.

But porn magazines have been on the shelves since before I reached my teens in the 1970s, and their covers have been subject to rigorous 'no nipple' rules for many years. The *Sunday Sport* has been around since 1986, and the *Daily Sport* since 1991. Lads' mags have been a staple offering since the 1990s. Furthermore, all of these publications, without exception, have seen their circulations decline steeply for years. If this is sexualisation, our high streets have been desexualised rather than sexualised in the past decade. What appears to have changed is an increasing conservatism in the British discourse.

Undaunted by the inconclusive results of this study, the *Guardian* followed up with further hysteria in an article by the normally level-headed Zoe Williams, headlined "The pornification of Britain's high streets".[39]

Pornification

It should be noted that pornification is a word invented by the anti-porn campaigner Gail Dines. Pornification takes the sexualisation concept to a new level, suggesting that pornography itself has seeped into every corner of our consciousness without us noticing.

Indeed, Zoe Williams says:

> However, in the past I've always thought that, because they made no dent on my consciousness, they didn't matter. What should have been obvious is that, like air pollution, just because you can't always see it, doesn't mean it's not poisonous.

Williams ignores the obvious difference: that even if poison is invisible to the eye, it can still be easily and unambiguously detected. So can Williams provide straightforward examples of pornification? Well... no. She talks about some of the photographs submitted, and provides some rambling quotes. But nothing that remotely backs her suggestion that pornification is real, measurable and getting worse. She closes the article by plugging Lose the Lads' Mags, a campaign front group created by Object and UK Feminista (groups to which the *Guardian* generously provides many column inches) before closing: "Look around now, though – outrage is building".

And she is right. I have watched the outrage build: among the handful of Object and UK Feminista activists and their supportive press, especially the *Guardian*, in parts of the Labour movement and other, smaller, left-wing organisations. The outrage was already there in the *Daily Mail*, and in the Conservative Party, but if anything has eased on the right as the left has increasingly taken over leadership of the anti-sex movement.

Polly Toynbee, Object and Mary Whitehouse

If any person perfectly encapsulates the left's swing from libertine to censorious, it is the veteran *Guardian* journalist Polly Toynbee. Toynbee is a commentator who writes on issues of social justice, inequality and child poverty. She comes into the porn-panic story in two eras, and two roles. In the 1970s, she was a member of the Williams Committee, mentioned previously, which examined the potential harms from pornography and decided none could be found; and when I spoke to her, Toynbee was Patron of Object.

In interviewing her for this book, I began by asking about the workings of the Williams Committee, and her involvement with it. She talked about the committee's work in sifting evidence for and against harm caused by pornography, and its conclusion that no evidence of harm had been presented.

She happily recalled the committee's encounters with the country's most prolific anti-porn campaigner:

> We had a wonderful time with Mary Whitehouse, who came several times, and said she could prove harm, because she had all these letters from wives who had been brutally abused, misused and had unreasonable things demanded of them by their husbands after reading pornography. So we said 'Well that's interesting. Can you show us some of these letters?' She said the letters were in boxes in her attic, and her husband had a bad back and couldn't get them down. So we said 'We'll send someone… to come and help you get the boxes down', and she avoided it, so we never got the letters, and we assumed they never really existed… so her evidence completely collapsed.

I was struck by the similarity between this description of Whitehouse's methods and the scare tactics adopted by Object, who claim to have spoken to victims of pornography, but seem incapable of providing their names or any other specifics.

When I asked Toynbee about her support for Object's censorship campaigns in comparison to her rejection of Mary Whitehouse's moralism, she was far vaguer, and her enthusiasm for evidence-based decision-making seemed to dissolve.

> I don't know, do they want outright banning? I think they want things taken from view more, don't they?... Lots of other things have happened... normalising of lap-dancing... the idea that ordinary businessmen – and taking business-women with them too – should be expected to think going to a lap-dancing club is normal. That didn't used to be the case, it was very much backstreet Soho peepshows, but it wasn't mainstream, it was naughty. And we were in favour of things being available if you wanted to be naughty and go and seek it out, but that's very different to having it in every high street.

I saw this as an odd position: strip clubs are OK in Soho but not close to home. They are fine when we accept them as naughty, but not when we think they are normal.

The Guardian's Pro-Censorship Role

The *Guardian* is a leading liberal newspaper, and has been at the forefront of breaking important news stories. The paper worked with *Wikileaks* to publish stories that exposed American war crimes in Iraq, and in 2013 broke the revelations, leaked by Edward Snowden, that the American and British governments were spying on their citizens as a matter of routine. It played a key role in exposing phone-hacking and police bribery within Rupert Murdoch's British newspaper business. It is fair to say that without the *Guardian*, at least some of these scandals may never have come to public attention. I have read the paper for years, both because of its high news quality, and to support a vital independent voice in the media.

However, the examples of sexual conservatism and censo-rious attitudes in the *Guardian* that have been outlined so far are not mere exceptions from its rule of high-quality journalism. The newspaper appears to have a blind spot over issues of sexual freedom, sexual commerce and sexual expression.

I first began to notice this in 2006. The UK adult entertainment industry was going through a 'growing up' spell. It had only emerged from the shadows of illegality a few years earlier, and was realising that it needed to professionalise and promote itself to the wider world. One of the effects of this change was the launch of an annual porn awards ceremony. Such things had taken place in Las Vegas and Berlin for years, but British pornographers were more used to keeping their profiles as low as possible, rather than openly promoting themselves.

The event took place in Hammersmith, West London, and the press were invited. The ceremony ran along the lines of any other awards-type event, although (having been organised by people with no previous experience of such a thing) was fairly error-prone – which added to the general sense of fun. Perhaps the pornstars handing out the trophies on stage should have been encouraged to stay sober until that part of the evening was over, but drunken awards ceremonies are hardly unique to the porn industry.

The *Guardian*'s coverage was never expected to be congratulatory, but the hatchet job it published, written by Paul Lewis, took many by surprise. The article was short, barely mentioned what happened at the ceremony, and took pleasure in sneering comments like: "strip away the innuendo, vulgar poses and exposed flesh, and it still seemed more like Confessions of a Window Cleaner, The Musical, than the Academy Awards".[40]

This was hardly surprising; perhaps it was too much to expect a highbrow publication, heavily staffed by Oxbridge graduates, to take such an event seriously. Indeed, it was not supposed to be a serious event. The comment does not seem entirely accurate though. "Vulgar poses and exposed flesh" seem to be part of many awards ceremonies, although what constitutes vulgarity is really down to the viewer's own attitudes. As for innuendo though? The porn industry hardly needs it. Innuendo is for those sections of the media that cannot openly and frankly talk about sex, meaning pretty much all of the media *except* the porn industry.

But the oddest part of the article was devoted to an interview with Gill Herd, the manager of a "nearby women's project", who (allegedly) told Lewis: "You can't possibly package porn as ordinary... At its essence it degrades women – violates and ojectifies [sic] them". Who is Gill Herd? What is the project she runs? What (specifically) are her issues with pornography? What is her expertise on the subject? Why did Lewis feel it was relevant to interview her, aside from the fact that she happened to be based 'nearby'? The article does not answer any of these questions. Searching for "gill herd women's project" on Google returns exactly one relevant link: Lewis's article. Do either Gill Herd or her project exist? I contacted Paul Lewis to ask these questions, but received no response.

What this illustrates is a classic piece of moral panickery, and a favorite *Guardian* tactic. Although the comment appears to be irrelevant to the overall article, it introduces the idea that pornography harms women, without exposing the journalist to the tiresome need of providing rationale or evidence to back the point. Pornography is juxtaposed with a concerned (perhaps imaginary) woman who is involved with some kind of women-related project. A casual reader will take away an implication of harm to women, although none is justified.

Over the following years, I saw far more coverage of this sort, and patterns began to emerge. What I initially took to be a combination of laziness and snobbery on the part of *Guardian* journalists appears to be an established editorial position on the part of the newspaper.

During the east London campaign to save strip venues, the stripper activists experienced the same dismissive and patronising responses from the *Guardian*. Invitations they sent to the paper's journalists were ignored, or resulted in similarly dismissive coverage. Requests by the activists to write columns putting their point of view were ignored (although Edie, Shelley and other activists are competent writers), while columns accusing strip clubs of exploiting, degrading and objectifying women were published on a regular basis.

For some years, the *Guardian* appeared to go out of its way to promote Object and UK Feminista. Despite the fact that both groups are tiny, and that many feminists are deeply opposed to their ideas, the pro-censorship version of feminism has been heavily promoted by the *Guardian*, and sex-positive voices, especially the voices of women in the sex industries, feature more rarely.

This behaviour is not exclusive to the *Guardian*, but it is particularly marked in the *Guardian's* case. The *Daily Mail* is expected to provide conservative reporting as a matter of routine, on subjects from sex to immigration to government economic policy. But in almost every subject area, other than sex, the *Guardian* demonstrates that it possesses the journalistic and editorial skills to address subjects honestly, and to spot the difference between fact and propaganda.

The *Guardian's* anti-sex campaign consists of regular articles linking porn to panic words including objectification, sexualisation, pornification, addiction, degradation and exploitation, along with occasional editorials in which it calls for censorship. This behaviour appears to be set by policy.

On 30th May 2013, the newspaper revealed its censorship hand, in an editorial titled "Internet pornography: Never again", which accused David Cameron of failing to lead in 'protecting children'. This was written in the wake of the murder of a child, April Jones, by a man who (it was claimed) had looked at 'violent pornography'. Linking a child murder to a moralistic cause is classic moral-panic behaviour. Child murders are thankfully rare, but sadly, they do happen intermittently, and are often exploited to underpin whatever the moral agenda of the day happens to be. There is no evidence that porn (violent or not) causes people to commit atrocities, any more than computer games or horror films do, but the hint is enough for the purposes of a moral panic. The editorial was riddled with the language of panic:

> Internet pornography is sometimes abusive and often violent... Violent pornography is easily and freely accessible, and at most requires only a credit card... The link between such material and actual violence, most commonly against women and children, is disputed [a rare moment of honesty – although "non-existent" would be more accurate]... But there is strong evidence that at the very least it is addictive, can normalise violence, and at the same time diminishes sympathy for its victims [dubious claims with no link or further evidence provided]... Abusive and violent pornography should be banned... the misery of the April Jones case should spur a revival of the effort [to censor pornography].

And so on, making claim after claim of harm, yet failing to mention that none of the allegations made are backed by any available research.

Why focus on the *Guardian* specifically? Because it plays a unique role in British life. It is trusted by its loyal readership for taking liberal positions, and for its commitment to honest journalism. Most readers have neither the time nor the will to independently verify every news article they read, so they decide which news outlets they trust. If a newspaper known for bravely exposing state and corporate crimes, and for the generally high quality of its journalism, is claiming porn causes harm – even that porn causes little girls to be murdered – then surely it must be true?

The reality – that the *Guardian* has taken a conscious decision to become a pro-censorship force – is hard to swallow. It took me, once a loyal Guardianista, several years to appreciate what was happening. For whatever reason (and I do not claim to understand the internal workings of the *Guardian*), a deeply conservative policy position has been adopted.

A clue is given by researcher and writer Dr Brooke Magnanti, who came to fame when she blogged about her life as a sex worker under the pseudonym Belle de Jour.

> After I won the *Guardian* Best British Weblog award in 2003, a number of female contributors to that paper suggested that if I was commissioned to write an article, they would quit. (In the end it was that bastion of Tory sensibility the *Telegraph* that offered me my first bylined article and first broadsheet column. Oh, the irony.)[41]

But perhaps it is not so ironic. Perhaps Magnanti, like myself and many others who considered ourselves to be on the progressive side of politics, had missed the shift that had taken place within the political left. We had not left the left, but the left had left us.

The Porn-Panic Winners

The fear business is a lucrative one, and so is highly competitive. In the more religious United States, tales of impending Armageddon are eagerly consumed, and Amazon is packed with titles such as *Are We Living in the End Times?*

The British are also avid consumers of fear, although in less religious forms. The media is in an almost constant state of panic over a variety of issues, and always on the lookout for new scare stories.

As the porn panic has grown in recent years, many figures have come forward as the prophets of doom, eager to sell their books and win speaking engagements. While Gail Dines has won plenty of the limelight, the media has sought out home-grown figures to become the faces of the pro-censorship lobby.

Object and UK Feminista emerged from a plethora of anti-sex feminist groups, and the leading figures of each group have increasingly been promoted as the British spokespeople for censorship. Julia Long of Object and Kat Banyard of UK Feminista both emerged from the scrum to be the spokespeople of the British anti-porn movement; each had her own book to sell. Both received generous coverage in the media as the panic grew in strength. Long's book, *Anti-Porn: The Resurgence of Anti-Pornography Feminism,* was published in 2012.

Certain UK newspaper editors worked hard to establish the two figures in the public mind, and one or the other seemed almost certain to take part in any televised discussion about pornography. Banyard appeared to be a particular favourite of the *Guardian,* which named her as "The UK's most influential young feminist"[42] in 2010, and regularly featured articles both about and written by her.

Although Mary Whitehouse's old organisation, now known as Mediawatch-UK, is still alive and well, its more overtly moralistic message tends to be eclipsed by the new, faux-liberal messages emerging from the puritanical left. Mediawatch-UK has responded by updating its language to an extent, borrowing ideas like objectification and sexualisation from anti-sex feminism, but the organisation is taken less seriously than it once was during Whitehouse's heyday.

Political Consensus

The anti-sex stances traditionally taken by the religious leaders, the Conservative Party and the right-wing press are now standard throughout the British media and British politics. The Labour Party has largely bought into the scare, and is competing with the Tories to be toughest on attacking sexual expression. Only the Liberal Democrats, and sometimes the Greens, show any scepticism over the need for more censorship.

The long view is that MacDworkinite, anti-sex feminism,

thwarted in its censorship goals in the United States by the First Amendment, has found a softer target in the UK, which has no First Amendment. Liberals, who have historically tended to resist censorship and anti-sex morality, have in the past been arguably more immune to moral panics than conservatives. If the same messages had come from Mary Whitehouse rather than Kat Banyard, from the *Daily Mail* rather than the *Guardian*, from the Tories rather than Labour, perhaps the left might have remained a more sceptical force when the state tried to impose Internet censorship. The appearance of Object and UK Feminista, and the presentation of these groups as representing mainstream feminism and women's rights, has done immense damage to the fight against censorship, and ensured that, from left to right of the political spectrum, the defence of free speech is almost non-existent.

The pieces of the porn-panic puzzle now fall into place. But the drive toward censorship is about far more than just pornography. The Internet threatens a myriad of vested interests, and its freedom is now under attack from every direction. We are in the throes of the Big Panic, and it appears to be getting worse.

6

The Big Panic

DON'T PANIC! – Douglas Adams, *The Hitchhiker's Guide to the Galaxy*

The 21st century in Britain has been marked by a rising tide of conservatism and moral panic. Old targets – porn and computer gaming for example – have been dusted off and attacked anew. To these have been added new threats to mankind (or more frequently, to 'women and children').

Moral entrepreneurs often deny that they want censorship, claiming instead that they merely seek to 'create debate on important issues'. But by claiming harm from various forms of expression, they wittingly or unwittingly create the conditions for censorship, and when censorship does actually follow the panic, they tend to be conspicuously absent in condemning it.

Moral entrepreneurs and state censors therefore work hand-in-hand, but maintain a distance: each side is best served by having, or having the appearance of having, little to do with the other. The censor is compromised if he is found involved in feeding moral panic that results in an increase of his own powers; likewise the moral entrepreneur is most effective while claiming to dislike censorship, but to be genuinely concerned about some supposed societal ill.

But by following the players carefully, one can see how intertwined these two interest groups can be. It is well known, for example, that the BBFC played a lobbying role during the video-nasties moral panic, and issued warnings about the dangers of uncensored horror videos; this, of course, eventually led to the BBFC itself being given a lucrative government monopoly as official censor of video. ATVOD played a very similar game while lobbying for its own powers to be enhanced. In 2014, the regulator issued a press release claiming (on the flimsiest evidential basis) that 44,000 children aged between 6 and 11 were watching porn each month[43]. The methodology used for calculating this number was so unreliable that the report included a line that effectively debunked itself:

> These demographics do not meet minimum sample size standards. Measures for these demographics may exhibit large changes month-to-month as a result and should be treated with caution.

ATVOD (which, it must be remembered, was supposed to be a government-approved regulator, not an anti-porn campaigning body) also convened a conference on 'child protection' in late-2013, which featured a scarcity of expertise in child protection. Instead the event featured anti-porn voices, including Object's Julia Long. I wrote to the organiser to point this out, and she responded flippantly:

> Thank you for your letter and suggestions for the joint ATVOD-QMUL conference on 12th December.
> We have finalised the composition of the panels and speakers. I'm familiar with the work of the speakers you suggest and have no doubt that they also have interesting contributions to make, perhaps at a different conference. Please let me know if you are organising such an event in the future.[44]

It is only thanks to media laziness that these links between state censors and freelance moral entrepreneurs, and their respective vested interests, are not explored more fully.

Later, the interests involved can be exposed at leisure, but by then it is too late. It is widely known now, three decades on, that 'video nasties' posed no threat to the moral health of the nation, and that the 'research' presented at the time was of little value; but to repeal the Video Recordings Act, which resulted from that moral panic, would take great political will. No politician would win many votes by making such a promise, so the law stays in place, along with the BBFC's censorship powers. Censorship is therefore a ratchet: very easy to advance, very hard to move backward. It took an entire century for the original Obscene Publications Act to be reformed, and its revised version is still in place today, even though it was widely seen as unnecessary 40 years ago.

The video-nasties moral panic played out over more than a year during 1983 and 1984, before culminating in the passage of the Video Recordings Act. In this new, digital era, moral panics can rise and fall in days, or even hours, and their architects have become skilled at lighting one fire after another. To attempt to expose moral panics (as I have done for the past few years) is therefore a repetitive game of whack-a-mole, and must be done in real-time as new panics pop up online.

But however effectively one combats moral panics, moral entrepreneurs are generally successful in sowing their seeds of doom. Most members of the public today have heard the porn-panic keywords repeated endlessly, and so believe that objectification, sexualisation, extreme porn, porn addiction and so on are real phenomena, and pose genuine threats. The debate is on the terms of the moral panic: porn is discussed in terms of its potential harms rather than its neutral or beneficial effects. And it really does not matter how interested or frightened the public actually is: during election campaigns, politicians will make promises that win votes, and if promising to 'protect children' will generate some positive headlines during a fraught campaigning cycle, so be it.

The porn panic was just one part of a broader social movement with the ultimate aim of making censorship acceptable. In the end, it would not matter which excuse was chosen to block Internet content: there are many ways to skin a cat. So long as it was established that free expression was dangerous, it mattered little whether the target was pornography or anything else.

The era of blaming everything bad on online expression – which I call the Big Panic – really began in the summer of 2011, when Britain's cities erupted in violence.

The British Riots

On a Thursday in August 2011, a young man called Mark Duggan was shot dead by police in Tottenham, north London. For two days, anger rose in Tottenham and beyond, until a Saturday-evening protest outside Tottenham police station turned violent. The rumour quickly propagated via text message and social media that a teenage girl had been assaulted by police at the protest (it is unclear whether this actually happened), and rioting began in inner-city areas across the country.

The police appeared to be slow to step in and take control. With some people emboldened by this, organised looting began. Although the early media coverage focused on anti-police rioting, within a day or so the focus shifted to the looters in various parts of the country, and genuine fear began to spread through the population. The scale of the violence was greatly exaggerated, and calls spread on social media for police to use weaponry – even live ammunition. When the police finally organised and fully deployed on Tuesday, the violence and looting fizzled out in hours.

Some rumours suggested that the police had been deliberately slow to deploy in order to send a message to the coalition government, which was planning heavy cuts to police budgets. Whatever the truth in that, the media began to demand that politicians explain what had happened, and do something about it. With some evidence that Blackberry's messenger (BBM), as well as Facebook and Twitter, had been used to organise rioting, the government found its culprit. The Prime Minister addressed Parliament on the issue. The *New York Times* quoted him:

"Everyone watching these horrific actions will be struck by how they were organized via social media," Mr. Cameron told Parliament during a special debate on the riots. "Free flow of information can be used for good. But it can also be used for ill. And when people are using social media for violence we need to stop them. So we are working with the police, the intelligence services and industry to look at whether it would be right to stop people communicating via these Web sites and services when we know they are plotting violence, disorder and criminality."[45]

During the unrest, the TV news channels had been pumping out repetitive riot coverage 24 hours a day, but were not blamed for the violence. Social media had been made the bogeyman, and would remain so. Although the Internet was well established, the rise of social media was a fairly recent phenomenon, and had democratised public discourse to an unprecedented level that posed a threat to politicians' and media corporations' ability to control the message.

The police apparently felt the same way, with the *Guardian* reporting a Metropolitan Police spokesman as saying that:

"really inflammatory, inaccurate" messages on Twitter were mainly to blame for the disorder. "Social media and other methods have been used to organise these levels of greed and criminality."[46]

Voices of reason were to be heard though. The Big Panic was young, and at this stage the media still sought out counter-opinions on such issues. Within government as well, free speech was defended. It later emerged that the Foreign Secretary William Hague had privately warned against censorship, pointing out that Britain could hardly lecture China or Arab states against repression while leaping to adopt the same repressive measures itself.[47]

As the Big Panic progressed, these voices of reason became increasingly muted. This first government suggestion of Internet censorship may have ruffled feathers, but as the scare stories became ever-more frequent, dissent faded and the need for censorship would eventually become broadly accepted as 'common sense'.

War on the First Amendment

Beneath the hysteria brought on by the riots, historic changes were taking place. The British state was losing control of its communications media. Telephones, mobile phones and SMS had always been operated within the jurisdiction of UK law. Police forces could order phones to be tapped, and could access people's call records and SMS messages. Intelligence services could – within the law or otherwise – intercept British people's communications.

But the new communications mechanisms were largely operated from overseas. Facebook and Twitter were American companies, as was Skype (acquired by Microsoft shortly before the riots), and RIM (the creator of Blackberry) was Canadian. Online email services such as Hotmail, Gmail and Yahoo! were all US-based. Strong encryption ensured that British users' private messages could not be easily accessed by UK authorities (although, as the NSA whistleblower Edward Snowden later revealed, the US and UK intelligence services had in fact gained access to vast amounts of private information via intimidation of service providers, or technical tricks).

For centuries, the UK had been able to ignore the US Constitution's First Amendment, which (to a large extent) guaranteed free speech to American citizens. Technology companies, faced with British government requests to provide a 'kill switch' to use during emergencies, could simply refuse, safe in the knowledge that they were protected by the US Constitution.

British authorities saw their powers of control seeping away, thanks to the globalising nature of the Internet, and they did not like that at all. Having resisted enshrining a strong commitment to free expression into British law for centuries, they now found it happening anyway.

Although the Big Panic had no single root cause, one of the reasons for it was undoubtedly a desire among the control-freak tendency of the British Establishment to shore up their declining powers. A clampdown on Internet free speech was coming, and while pornography was seen as a good excuse for this, in reality it had very little to do with porn. The right to view porn is simply harder to defend than the right to free speech, and so attacking porn is more fruitful than attacking other forms of expression. Britain's worthy defenders of civil liberty would be almost silent when Internet blocking was eventually proposed, because of squeamishness about defending sexual expression, and a fundamental contradiction between the supposedly liberal values and sexual prudishness of the new left.

And so the war on social media was underway. Unlike Facebook, which took care to preserve itself as a 'family-friendly' service, Twitter maintained a strong commitment to free expression, and so became a focus for the rage of a wide variety of prudes and censors.

The War on Twitter

Many of my more sexually liberated friends on Facebook often found themselves repeatedly censored due to Facebook's ultra-tight policies against nudity and sexual expression. Even images that were probably not in breach of policy would sometimes be removed by Facebook: one assumes that the team responsible for policing content does not have a great deal of time to spend examining each image before deciding whether to remove it. Once Facebook has issued a certain number of warnings for breaching policy, entire accounts can be removed. So it was unsurprising that pornstars, strippers, sex workers and others abandoned Facebook for the freer service, Twitter, where they could post explicit comments and images without fear of censorship.

Nobody on Twitter is forced to see anything they don't want to: anybody can unfollow or block accounts that offend them. But censors exist to restrict *other* people from seeing things they dislike, and so Twitter naturally became hated by control freaks, both amateur and professional. An anti-Twitter backlash was brewing.

The first hint of a state response came in 2010, when Paul Chambers (who planned to go on holiday a week later) sent the following tweet after a local airport announced its closure due to bad weather:

> Crap! Robin Hood airport is closed. You've got a week and a bit to get your shit together otherwise I'm blowing the airport sky high!!

The famously dry British sense of humour failed the authorities, and Chambers was arrested for sending a 'menacing' message, which is illegal under the Communications Act of 2003. Not only did the preposterous case come to court, but Chambers was found guilty. It took three appeals, as well as publicity built up with the help of the comedian Stephen Fry, before Chambers was eventually cleared.

There could be no sensible security justification for the 'Twitter joke trial', as it became known. As with the law criminal-ising the possession of 'extreme porn', the authorities were trying to get a handle on the free-speech 'problem' by intimidation: making an example of an individual. The message was clear: tweet at your peril. On the surface, the case backfired, making the state a laughing stock at home, and the whole country a joke worldwide. But it was likely that British Twitter users were a little more careful to self-censor from then on. The authorities would also be more careful to ensure their next targets were less sympathetic figures.

Meanwhile, amateur censors would have to content themselves with trying to censor Twitter on a small scale. The service provided a facility for reporting spam, so that fake accounts could be quickly identified and closed down. Activists of all political stripes quickly realised that they could use this feature against their online enemies. Twitter's algorithms would try to identify spam accounts – presumably based on the assumption that a relatively new account with few followers, but lots of complaints, only existed for spam purposes. A small but well-organised group could report genuine accounts as spam, and get them closed down. I initially saw this happen to some atheist and pro-life accounts based in the US, and it was not uncommon to receive a tweet from a new account along the lines: "My old account @xyz was closed down – please follow this one".

The Block Bot

Inevitably, somebody with more technical ability than love for free expression had the idea of automating this mass-blocking activity. An amorphous movement known as Atheism Plus had tried to create a somewhat strange blend of atheism with political ideas such as feminism and anti-racism. From Atheism Plus emerged the Block Bot, a British creation that grouped 'bad' Twitter accounts into three levels of terribleness. By simply installing the Block Bot, a Twitter user could automatically block all of the accounts listed by the Bot at level one (the 'worst of the worst'), level two or level three (those that might offend one's great-grandma if she had a hangover). The Block Bot's website explained as follows:

> The Block Bot is a Twitter application to automatically block the people added to its lists. Once installed, it works in the background, discreetly blocking them on your Twitter account.
>
> The Block Bot can be used anonymously, and makes no change whatsoever to your Twitter profile. The blocks are made silently, and (from the point of view of the person being blocked) are indistinguishable from ordinary blocks. You may follow @TheBlockBot Twitter account if you wish, but there is no requirement to do so.
>
> The Block Bot was created specifically for the atheist feminist community and currently includes a strong contingent of transgender social-justice activists and intersectional feminists. It should go without saying that blockers, as with any other human beings, make assessments based on their own perspectives and world-view and any commentary they make is their own. Blockers do not make judgments based on a set rubric, but make complex decisions based on a variety of factors in an attempt to serve our subscribers as best they can.

As somebody who abhors state-imposed censorship, I find it inexplicable that anyone would choose to censor their *own* view of the world voluntarily: the three wise monkeys come to mind, although there is nothing wise about deliberately closing one's ears and eyes to reality. I have very occasionally blocked people on Twitter if they repeatedly targeted me with annoying messages, but have had no other reason to do so. I dislike racism and other forms of bigotry, but I have no fear that I might see a racist tweet and become a racist myself, or fly into some uncontrollable, all-consuming rage upon reading one (I would either challenge or unfollow somebody who sent racist tweets though – I have little interest in seeing them). I accept that bad things can be said, and I can challenge, observe or ignore those things as I choose.

The Block Bot must have come from the deepest sense of superiority, arrogance and elitism: the belief that one has the right to tell *other* people which ideas they should or should not see. This applies to all censors: only a true elitist could try to dictate which ideas other people have access to, rather than join the debate and win by the force of reason. Or perhaps, alternatively, it originates from the deepest feelings of insecurity: a knowledge that one's beliefs are so weak and frail that opposing ideas would win in a fair debate, and so must be crushed.

What kind of people would install the Block Bot, and thereby block Twitter accounts they had never even heard of? Presumably people with no original ideas, people desperate to follow others, and people lacking confidence in their own political beliefs to such a degree that they fear *bad ideas* might somehow enter and infect their fragile little minds.

All censorship is subject to mission creep. Once a mechanism exists, it puts power into somebody's hands, and power always corrupts. Even if one accepts that sexism, racism and online abuse are good excuses for censorship, does one trust the Block Bot's custodians to always impartially apply objective rules? Is it even *possible* to objectively define what is racist or sexist?

As if to validate the point that nobody can be trusted with powers of censorship, the Block Bot began to blacklist people who could in no way be called bigots or abusers: some of them apparently blocked for daring to challenge the Block Bot's self-appointed censorship mission. According to a report at breitbart.com[48], the science writer Richard Dawkins has been listed – and Dawkins is certainly reputed for being a somewhat shrill Twitter-user at times; but so has the mild-mannered physicist, science writer and broadcaster Brian Cox. Blocked accounts have included those of journalists and – most tellingly – parodies. Never let it be said that censorship and humour are compatible.

Witch-hunting is an old human activity. Centuries ago, the cry of 'witch' was enough for the mob to lynch somebody. In 1950s America, the accusation of being 'communist' or 'homosexual' was enough to ruin careers and lives, whether true or not. And in today's post-liberal era, an accusation of being a 'sexist', 'racist' or 'homophobe' is enough to permanently stigmatise somebody, regardless of how true it is.

The Block Bot is an illustration of how, in today's Britain, the greatest attacks on free speech have increasingly come from the political left, whereas they once came from the right. Or to look at this from a different angle: fascism changes its clothing to suit the era. Because liberal ideas and values triumphed in earlier decades, it is natural that fascist behaviours today would appear cloaked in language once associated with liberalism. There is nothing progressive about censorship; there is no such thing as a 'progressive censor'.

So it was unsurprising that the next attack by the state on Twitter users would come shrouded in 'liberal' attitudes that would attract public support, rather than derision.

War on 'Misogynistic Twitter Trolls'

Catching up with an old school friend in early-2014 and making general small-talk, I was surprised when he asked me: "What about these Twitter trolls then?" My friend, a financial adviser, was never much interested in technology, and yet here he was using a word once only known to hard-core geeks like myself. 'Troll' is an old term used by the online community to refer to people who make deliberately provocative posts on forums in order to disrupt discussions and stir up animosity. Those who rise to such provocation are generally reminded to not 'feed the troll' by responding to them.

The fact that my friend was using the term was a sign that it had entered mainstream discourse (though, as is usually the case, its meaning had become twisted in the process). The story that brought trolling into the mainstream was that of Caroline Criado-Perez, a journalist, who had lent her support to an online campaign to feature a woman on the new £5 banknote.

According to a journalist friend who watched events unfold, Criado-Perez had come in for pointless and sometimes very nasty abuse from a handful of people on Twitter. So far, so unsurprising: 'armchair warriors' are legion online, and always have been. People who are shy and retiring in real life become infinitely braver when they're anonymous and far away from their victim. As a veteran of online political discourse myself, I've been threatened with death before, and called pretty much every name imaginable. While this can be an unpleasant experience first time round, it is important to remind oneself that nobody intending to actually do harm to anyone will make their intentions known, publicly, in advance. Given that users are easily traceable (unless they have very good technical knowledge), and that making threats online is a crime in the UK, to do such a thing is a sign of nothing more than stupidity.

Criado-Perez was the perfect victim: female, white, blonde and middle-class. Some of the tweets she received were alleged to contain rape threats: now the long-awaited opportunity for an anti-Twitter panic had arrived. Although earlier generations of feminists had been strident in their insistence that women should be treated equally, rather than infantilised and offered special treatment, the mainstream feminist message has subtly morphed to embrace the opposite position. Abuse of women online is falsely held up as evidence of unacceptable misogyny, while abuse of men (which studies suggest is, in fact, more common) appears to offend no group in particular. The old, patriarchal idea that women (and especially young, pretty women) are the 'weaker sex', and need special protection, is now a mainstream feminist message.

Armed with Criado-Perez's photograph, the media went into moral-panic overdrive. 'Abusive Twitter trolls' and 'misogynistic trolls' made the headlines. Arrests were quickly made, and the media campaign continued unrelentingly for several months. For those caught unaware by the reporting, it must have seemed as though 'Twitter abuse' and 'Internet trolls' had just appeared out of nowhere: the implication being that a platform allowing free speech was somehow making previously nice people into dangerous animals, so proving that unregulated free speech is unacceptable.

A Something-Must-Be-Done moment arrived. A kneejerk campaign quickly consolidated around the idea of a Twitter button to report abuse. An inevitable petition was launched calling on Twitter to add an 'abuse' button, although what Twitter was supposed to do with allegedly abusive tweets was not specified. To have a team of people appointed to look at countless tweets and decide what is abusive, and if so how abusive, whether the abuse is somehow warranted, whether it is satirical or a parody, would be impossible to do effectively without losing passionate debate and bad-taste humour in the process.

Twitter already provided two useful functions for such cases: the first was retweet. A problem shared with a friend is a problem halved. A problem shared with hundreds or thousands of Twitter followers is rapidly dispensed with. The second is the block button; abuse is hard to ignore, but nobody on Twitter is required to read tweets from anyone they do not want to. When I have been genuinely angered or upset by online comments – for example, because I am Jewish, Holocaust jokes have occasionally been directed at me – there are several things I can do. The least satisfying is to respond angrily. Better is to ignore. Better still is to respond with humour. If that is not possible, I can retweet, and allow others to respond. This is therapeutic, because it reminds me that I am not alone, and that the abuser is the minority. It is also, in my experience, far more uplifting to know that the community can deal with an idiot, and that we have no need for higher authorities – whether police, Block Bot or Twitter's abuse team – to fight our battles for us. Finally, I can block – although as mentioned, I have almost never found the need to do so.

Catering to the Most Sensitive

The Criado-Perez incident brings to mind Ofcom's TV-censorship regime. A programme may be watched by millions, but a tiny number of complaints – even just one can be enough – is taken by the censor as evidence of public discontent. The most sensitive in society set the standards for everybody else. The same system works in ATVOD's regulation of online video, and in the censorship of advertising by the Advertising Standards Authority.

Eventually, two individuals, a young man and a young woman, stood trial for abusing Criado-Perez. By the time of the trial, the media had apparently forgotten the 'torrent' and 'barrage' of horrific abuse that had earlier been reported, and accepted that two scapegoats would be enough. The prosecution told the court that "Caroline Criado-Perez has suffered life-changing psychological effects from the abuse which she received on Twitter".

That being the case, one must sympathise for the journalist; she is clearly a person of particularly sensitive disposition. Thankfully though, she recovered quickly enough, and even used her newfound fame to build a public profile as a journalist and feminist activist.

This may well be unfair to Criado-Perez herself: prosecutors invariably exaggerate the effects of crimes, in order to get harsh sentences. That, after all, is their job.

The pair of 'Twitter trolls' – Isabella Sorley, 23 and John

Nimmo, 25 – were found guilty, and sentenced to 12 weeks and 8 weeks in jail, respectively. The two cut pathetic figures: both overweight and unattractive, their photographs were happily plastered across the news media alongside those of the slim and pretty Criado-Perez. Sorley had 21 previous convictions for being drunk and disorderly, but the likelihood she was a depressed alcoholic was not mentioned.

The fact that the worst of the abusers was a woman was also inconvenient, given the 'torrent of online misogyny' narrative that had developed. Criado-Perez later said that Sorley had been raised in a "society steeped in misogyny", and so was conditioned to hate women.[49] This is what tends to be referred to as a 'feminist analysis'. As with religious 'reasoning', the conclusion of such an analysis is decided in advance – misogyny – then evidence is cherry-picked to fit this outcome. It seems highly unlikely that Sorley's motivation was, in fact, that she hated Criado-Perez because of her gender, but in the age of dumbed-down identity politics, such explanations are easy and fashionable, and the true reasons are generally more complex and less gratifying.

In fact, the trial coverage reeked of sneering class snobbery. The greatest impetus for censorship tends to come where unacceptable lines are crossed, and there is no line more fiercely defended by the middle classes than that between themselves and the unwashed masses. Before the birth of the digital network, the middle classes could be confident that they could maintain their distance from the lower classes – and they have always gone out of their way to do so, by choosing where to work, live, eat, drink, dance, holiday, educate their children and so on. The Internet, and specifically social media, created an unprecedented space in which the likes of Isabella Sorley might encounter someone like Caroline Criado-Perez. No wonder the journalistic and political classes have become so obsessed with the problem of 'Internet trolls'.

But the coverage largely ignored the vital question of whether people should be jailed for causing offence. Is it the job of the law to censor public discourse in order to cater for the needs of the most easily offended? Certainly, we as a society have become far less tolerant of unpleasant behaviour in the past couple of decades, and have elevated things that were once merely seen as annoying to the level of total unacceptability.

Behind the scenes, prosecutions for 'trolling' have increased sharply. In 2004, the year after 'malicious communications' were criminalised by the Communications Act, 143 people were convicted. By 2014, the number had risen to 1,209.[50] When the Labour opposition has had anything to say about this, it has typically been to accuse the government of 'doing too little, too late'. In November 2014, the Labour MP John Mann went further, suggesting a complete Internet ban for 'trolls'.[51] This would be akin, in the pre-Internet age, to sealing a person's mouth and eyes shut if they said mean things to people in public. When it comes to free speech, there has been a virtual absence of intelligent political debate, no word of caution about rising authoritarianism, or about the slippery slope of censorship. Parliamentarians, backed by political activists and journalists from across the political spectrum, appear to be engaged in a race to the bottom. Security and the 'online safety' of women and children have come to not only trump liberty, but entirely sideline it.

Free Speech and Identity Politics

Free speech, once the bedrock of liberalism, has – quite literally – become a dirty word on the political left. For a while in 2014, it even became fashionable for some online activists to mock the defence of free speech as FREEZEPEACH, using the argument that free speech cannot be allowed while some groups remain oppressed. The argument is a circular one, because in the swamp of identity politics, some groups are deemed to be permanently oppressed, by definition. So the argument goes: all women are oppressed; all men are privileged; therefore men cannot have free speech, because they use it to oppress women.

This new definition of privilege and oppression is strange indeed. Certainly, in my activism days, we campaigned endlessly to support oppressed groups. But then, oppression was something that *happened* to you. So for example, the theft of Palestinian land in the West Bank was (and remains) a clear-cut instance of the oppression of a group of people: namely Arabs living in the West Bank. In the intervening years, oppression (at least, as used by the left) has become something entirely different. Now, oppression is something you *are*. So a person can have a happy, healthy childhood, access to education and healthcare, be well fed for their entire life and have a well-paid career, but if they happen to check certain identity boxes, they are automatically deemed oppressed, and so (and here the reasoning becomes contorted in the extreme) they must have additional privileges to balance their oppression. In other words, the more oppressed someone is said to be, the more privilege they must have.

The new counter-Enlightenment does not just reject Liberty; it necessarily attacks Equality, which half a century ago was a non-negotiable bedrock of left-wing politics.

Thus, oppression has transformed from something nobody would wish upon themselves, to something everybody wants. I first became aware of this on seeing a tweet by a black lesbian from London, who wrote about her 'oppressions'. Having three oppressions, it seems, is license to tell other people to shut up on the basis that (in this case) they may be white, male, straight or (horror!) all three.

So we find ourselves in a looking-glass world where people want to claim oppression, and then use their oppression to censor other people who are privileged. There is perhaps no better example of the deep intellectual decline of the left than this doublethink. Someone can be silenced merely for their gender, sexuality, race or other arbitrary aspect of their identity: again, the new left and the far-right become virtually interchangeable. Both stand firmly opposed to solidarity or unity, and instead seek to divide society into arbitrary, opposing groups.

The Big Panic provided an apparently endless list of examples of this 'oppression as excuse for censorship' phenomenon. People who had never personally suffered anything that could truly be called oppression were now self-labelling as oppressed and turning their righteous anger against any form of expression that upset them. And the mainstream left stood by and watched, or positively cheered from the side-lines as the lust for censorship grew.

One particularly worrying example was the 2014 closure of an art exhibition, Exhibit B, at the Barbican in London following a fairly small protest. Even a decade earlier, it would have been hard to envisage wholesale bans on art taking place in Britain, let alone supported by many 'progressives'. But now, because the protesters in question were black, and were claiming the work to be racist, the gallery rolled over and a huge act of censorship was allowed to take place. Here was oppression-as-privilege in action: one cannot imagine that the gallery or police would allow an exhibition to be closed by a crowd of far-right skinheads or fundamentalist Christians. The public would cheer as police batons cracked white skulls to ensure the gallery remained open to the public. Yet here, an estimated hundred protesters were deemed privileged enough to censor art in the British capital, precisely because they were 'oppressed'.

Exhibit B showed a Human Zoo: black actors in poses that represented the worst evils of African colonialism and slavery. It had received five-star reviews in other cities, and was stoutly defended by the actors themselves. The protesters (as well as supporters I discussed the issue with) happily admitted they had not seen the exhibition, but felt they did not need to: they could censor simply because it featured black people representing a horrific era in black history. This argument closely mirrors the feminist claim of "I am female and therefore have the right to suppress images of other women". Every discussion I had on the issue ultimately came down to simple racism: the artist (Brett Bailey) was white, so had no right to depict certain things, however well he might have done it; and the audience too would be largely white, and so had no right to see black suffering depicted. To turn the reasoning around exposes the fascistic intent: for example, to deny a black artist the right to depict the Irish potato famine on the basis that only white people starved to death would not be accepted anywhere.

The Ethiopian-British poet Lemn Sissay was a rare black voice against censorship. He made the point that the more horrific an event, the more important it is to remember it:

> If I had children I would take them to see this exhibition too. "daddy did this really happen?" they would ask through tears "yes" I would reply. And our conversations would be elevated to why it happened and how it kinda happens today.[52]

Mob calls for censorship are nothing new; the fact that 'liberal' society is now inclined to stand aside and tolerate the mob, because the mob is black, or female, or gay, or trans, is the frightening new reality.

The idea that public discourse should be censored to suit the needs of small numbers of sensitive people increasingly came to the fore during the Big Panic. Meanwhile, the attacks on pornography became more generalised, and were turned against even the softest forms of sexual expression. A series of campaigns appeared, as if by magic, each one based on the false idea that any sexual expression is automatically sexist, and therefore offensive to women (some women, anyway), and must be suppressed.

Most of the campaigns were created by existing anti-sex groups. Each was astroturf: designed to look like grassroots. Small numbers of dedicated activists, with the help of social media and tame journalists, contrived to create the appearance of a mass movement. Feminism, which half a century earlier had fought for female liberation, was now mobilised for the purpose of attacking and destroying all representations of the female body in the public sphere.

7

The Suppression of the Female Body

I think on-stage nudity is disgusting, shameful and damaging to all things American. But if I were 22 with a great body, it would be artistic, tasteful, patriotic, and a progressive religious experience – Shelley Winters

A creation of Object and UK Feminista in 2013, Lose the Lads' Mags set out to get lads' mags removed from supermarkets. The campaign claimed that lads' mags are "sexist, harmful and can breach equality law". As usual, the claims of harm were never backed by any evidence; the mention of equality law is reminiscent of the failed attempt by the MacDworkinites to ban pornography using US civil-rights legislation. The Lose the Lads' Mags website explained:

New legal advice obtained by UK Feminista and Object reveals that displaying these publications can constitute sexual harassment or sex discrimination under the Equality Act 2010. Employees could take action on this basis and, where the magazine is visibly on display, customers could also have a claim.[53]

Along with the (unlikely) threat of legal action against super-markets, small groups of anti-sex activists picketed individual stores. Quickly, the Co-operative supermarket caved in to the morality campaigners, and insisted that lads' mags must be sold in 'modesty bags' – or 'burqas' as some anti-censorship commen-tators quipped.

Not all feminists saw the attack on lads' mags as a pro-female campaign. The stripper and sexual-freedom activist Edie Lamort wrote an impassioned letter to the Co-op's Chief Executive:

> As a woman I find the current trend towards more puritan
> values very disturbing. Lobby groups such as UK Feminista
> and Object represent the more extreme and fanatical end of
> this trend and I am very disappointed that the Co-op has
> buckled under pressure from them. With the... general moral
> panic at the moment about 'sexualisation' this is another
> retrograde step. It is almost like we are experiencing a sexual
> counter-revolution.
>
> I am worried about this overall message that demonises
> the female body and buys into centuries old patriarchal
> tradition that female flesh is sinful and corrupting. It is this
> mentality that spurred the Witch Trials of the 16th Century
> and in more recent times has cast a veil of silence over sexual
> abuse. It leads to an environment where people are made to
> feel shame about a perfectly natural urge leading to anger and
> frustration rather than self-awareness and understanding.
>
> The message the Co-operative is sending out is that it
> agrees with the backward idea that female sexuality and the
> female body is essentially a corrupting and bad thing and
> therefore must be hidden. That the female body is dirty,
> wrong, and bad. It is also extremely hypocritical as celebrity
> magazines such as *OK* and *Heat* are far more salacious and
> negative about bodies...
>
> We have come along way since the 60s, and the emanci-
> pation of all of us to wear what we like (a woman will not
> longer be branded 'tart' for wearing a short skirt) and to
> explore our sexual selves, which has been a very important
> social force. I can guarantee you that if this trend towards
> puritanism continues we will see a rise in sexual harassment,
> sexual assault and rape. This is because the message you and
> others are sending is that sex and especially of the female
> kind is inherently wrong. This will make zealots more

confident about chastising the 'temptress' or slut-shaming women who dare to be emancipated. The train of thought that goes 'oh she's a slut look at her she deserved it' will be encouraged by actions such as modesty bags.[54]

Despite the repeated claim that society was becoming 'sexualised', and that lads' mags provided firm evidence of that, the genre was already in steep decline. *Nuts* magazine had launched in 2004, and peaked at over 300,000 sales in 2005, but by late-2013 had declined over 80% from its high point.[55] Following Co-op's 'modesty bag' decision, *Nuts'* editor, Dominic Smith, decided to pull the magazine from sale in that chain. Within a few months, the magazine's publisher decided to close the title. Among dozens of women's titles (many of which featured paparazzi shots of celebrity cellulite and other bullying attacks on women's bodies), only one weekly men's title, *Zoo*, now remained.

No More Page 3

Of all the pro-censorship campaigns of the Big Panic, one stands out as cleverer, and far more successful, than all the rest.

According to a campaign representative I encountered during a university debate, No More Page 3 was born during the 2012 London Olympics. Following 'Super Saturday', when 12 British athletes won gold medals, the campaign's founder Lucy-Anne Holmes was (purportedly) angered when she saw that the space given to a picture of medal-winning athlete Jessica Ennis in the *Sun* was less than that given to the topless Page-3 model.

It is a clever campaigning position, pitting tabloid-style national pride in Our Jessica against a topless image, but scratch the surface and it becomes meaningless. There is no doubt that the *Sun*, which is prided for its sports coverage (if little else) devoted vast acreage of paper to the medal winners on that day. Of the dozen gold medalists, the biggest hero of the day was Mo

Farrah, who won three golds and probably attracted the most image space in the press.

The underlying claim is that the Page-3 model was somehow being treated as more important than Jessica Ennis. It contrasts two women with each other, for no reason other than they are both women, and draws a conclusion that nobody would take seriously if they thought for long about it. After all, the *Sun*'s TV guide on that day would also have taken up more space than Ennis' picture, but nobody would claim for a moment that the newspaper thought the TV schedule was more important than her sporting achievement.

But yes, it was clever, and the kind of primitive non-argument that will feed into mob mentality. One can imagine a far-right group making a similar point if – say – a picture of a Muslim preacher received more space than a picture of a poppy on Remembrance Sunday. In fact, this kind of meaningless, rabble-rousing argument is the very kind of thing one expects from the *Sun* newspaper itself. So while we can applaud the campaign for its creativity, it is obvious on reflection what Holmes' problem is: not that an unknown woman was given more space than Ennis, but that a *topless* woman was.

The argument is thus an old morality one wrapped in a thin feminist veneer – "how disgraceful that a woman should get more acclaim for showing her breasts than for winning a gold medal!" – which is not, of course, what happened.

Holmes' smartest move was in her selection of target. In picking on the *Sun*, of all publications, she was attacking what is certainly the most polarising publication in the UK, with a history of inaccurate, biased, bullying and bigoted reporting. She had pinpointed the exact instance of sexual expression that would attract the broadest possible opposition.

In order to build support to the maximum extent possible, the campaign initially took pains to distance itself from more overtly anti-sex campaigners, and to insist that it had no problem with sexual expression, except for the very specific instance of breasts in newspapers. As if to demonstrate that it were not a sour-faced, prudish movement, it selected the slightly odd campaign slogan: "Boobs Aren't News". One might note that most of what appears in a modern newspaper is not news, from travel guides and TV reviews to recipes and horoscopes. But the oversimplified, childlike arguments and slogans were perfect for transforming the anti-sex movement from a small, extreme-sounding clique moaning circle into a mass phenomenon that could attract the support of the wholesome girls and ladies of Middle England.

But in the months following the campaign's launch, the cheerful 'we love sex, honest!' mask slipped. No More Page 3 representatives attended Gail Dines' London Stop Porn Culture launch conference in 2014: a strange choice for a body that had no problems with sexual expression beyond one carefully chosen example. From its original insistence that it had no links with the anti-sex movement, it shifted its position until it formed a bridge between existing anti-sex activists and mainstream campaigners. This was a powerful position to be in.

By focusing on the fact that children might easily see Page 3, and combining that with anti-Murdoch noises (the *Sun*'s owner is almost universally disliked), No More Page 3 created a base that ranged from trade unions to girl guides. Based on individual encounters I had, online and offline, it was clear that the movement also attracted religious support, but this was carefully played down. Religious morality does not play well in Britain (or: "We don't do religion", as one of Tony Blair's advisers once put it to a journalist trying to probe into Blair's personal beliefs).

No More Page 3 made itself sound so eminently reasonable that it even divided pro-pornography activists. I came to realise how carefully it had pitched itself when one woman, who had vociferously opposed the government ban on 'rape porn', expressed herself fully in favour of removing Page 3 from the *Sun*. I probed her reasoning, but it did not appear to extend beyond "boobs aren't news" or "but kids might see it".

No More Page 3 spokespeople were trained to insist, no matter what, that they did not want censorship. But to demand (sorry, request – it truly was the politest of campaigns) the removal of content from a newspaper could be described as nothing else. In common with many pro-censorship movements, No More Page 3 insists on the narrowest possible definition of censorship: that resulting from law. But a censor can also be defined as "any person who supervises the manners or morality of others", a description that perfectly describes the campaign, which – we can safely assume – is not primarily made up of *Sun* readers.

The discussion of harm was handled in the same, slippery way. When I debated against No More Page 3 at Loughborough University, the spokesperson insisted that the campaign had *never* claimed to have evidence that Page 3 was harmful; and yet the remainder of her points were devoted to talking about objectification, body-image issues, rape culture, sex addiction and the other standard porn-panic talking points. Their argument boiled down to: "We're not claiming it's harmful, but just *look* at all the harm it's causing!"

Were I ever to create a parody of an anti-sex campaign, it would look something like the FAQ on No More Page 3's website[56], which was packed with moments of amusement, and many head-scratching ones. Its statement on censorship appeared not to understand the meaning of the word: "NMP3 isn't asking for censorship... NMP3 is asking, politely that page 3 be removed voluntarily" – as if the addition of 'politely' and 'voluntarily' would somehow change the meaning of the word 'censorship'. Would far-right nationalism become more acceptable if it 'politely' asked foreigners to 'voluntarily' leave the country at the earliest opportunity? Apparently so: fascists, take note!

Perhaps the weirdest sentence on the page compared women

who show their breasts with men who black-up: "Page 3… mocks and disrespects women just like racist features like the black and white minstrel show and gollywogs [sic] used to mock people of colour". Inadvertently and repeatedly, the campaigners made clear their disgust, not for sexism, but for the women who let the side down by allowing their breasts to be seen in public.

In attracting so many people to its cause, No More Page 3 did more harm to free expression than any other campaign, for a simple reason: by finding one single case where censorship of the female body was widely accepted, they created the precedent that the unclothed female body *can* be harmful; and this was all the pro-censorship movement needed. Once one case was accepted, then the general case must be accepted: if female nudity can be harmful in one context, it can be harmful in others contexts too. No More Page 3 created the conditions for the slippery slope towards censorship that the rest of the morality movement had largely failed to do.

Sexualised Music Videos

As the anti-sex movement targeted softer content with a Think-Of-The-Children message, it was inevitable that music videos would come under attack. The Bailey Review on sexualisation had singled out music videos as a problem (although, as previously mentioned, it had not carried out any actual research into potential harm, but simply polled parental attitudes).

Since their invention, music videos had come under fire from morality campaigners, but this was a phenomenon better known in the United States, with its powerful Christian right, than in Britain. Many of the attacks on popular music in America contained thinly-veiled racism. US society was racially segregated for most of its history, until relatively recently, and most white Americans had had little contact with black Americans or their cultures, until the rise of music recording and radio. Although black artists were often boycotted by radio stations, white performers, from Elvis Presley onwards, began to copy black music, and young white people began to dance to it. Unsurprisingly, this infuriated white conservatives.

A 1960s circular from the Citizens Council of Greater New Orleans reads as follows:

Help Save The Youth of America
DON'T BUY NEGRO RECORDS
(If you don't want to serve negroes in your place of business, then do not have negro records on your jukebox or listen to negro records on the radio.)

The screaming, idiotic words, and savage music of these records are undermining the morals of our white youth in America.

Don't Let Your Children Buy, or Listen To These Negro Records...[57]

Such a message shows more than hatred or anger: it reveals fear. As well as breaching the carefully constructed walls of racial segregation, black music and dance had caused a deeper concern: it was highly sexual. African dance had always been more 'wild' than the European equivalent. Now, as civil rights and anti-colonialism movements peaked, and segregation ended, continents were belatedly colliding. For the first time, black music entered mainstream Western culture. The dam broke. This was not a meeting of equals: African culture poured over white society like a tsunami.

Blues, jazz and rock and roll had just been the beginning. Now soul, hip hop, disco, reggae, dancehall, afrobeat, soca, dub, house, R&B and many other genres sold records by the millions and entered the charts worldwide. By the turn of the century, it was hard to find music in the British charts that did not have some black roots.

And the videos that came with the music showed another

African influence: clothing became skimpier, hips and backsides rolled in a way that white bodies had never before moved. As the moral panic against 'sexualised' music videos took root, it was not just a reaction to music; it was a reaction to black music.

Black female artists came under particular attack during the Big Panic. Especially singled out for criticism were Beyoncé, Rihanna and Nicki Minaj. But far from apologise and cover themselves up, all three of these artists revelled in their displays of sexuality, and responded to attacks by becoming more 'sexualised', apparently taking enjoyment from taunting the mostly white, middle-class commentators that were attacking them. Beyoncé's famous performance outfits became more revealing. Rihanna turned up to the 2014 Council of Fashion Designers Awards in a near-transparent dress, which generated an inevitable barrage of outrage. Minaj's *Anaconda* video gave the finger to her critics, being a celebration of her famously rounded backside, and featuring the line, delivered as a parody of a prissy, white girl: "Oh. My. Gosh. Look at her BUTT!"

Prudish anger mounted, with article headlines such as "Don't call Beyonce's sexual empowerment feminism"[58] trying to create a faux-liberal case for demanding that the singers cover themselves up. But there was no contest: three of the world's most confident and talented black female performers could easily handle whatever the bloggers and journalists could dish out. Commentators were reduced to whining, inaccurately and patronisingly, that the singers were the 'victims' of a white, male-dominated capitalist music machine. The women, and their millions of fans, paid little attention.

Given how deeply rooted the Big Panic was in the political left, and that the anti-sex movement was dominated by white, middle-class women, endless overt attacks on black performers would begin to look suspiciously racist. A white target for the rage was needed. Enter Miley Cyrus.

Cyrus had committed multiple sins in the eyes of moralists.

She had been a child star, and now had the nerve to grow up and become an attractive young woman. She appeared naked in the video for her single *Wrecking Ball*, and, most outrageous of all, during a 2013 live TV performance, she *twerked*.

Although twerking was a fairly new term, it described a dance move that had been around for decades, if not centuries. Nobody who has seen videos for hip hop, dancehall, R&B or other black music styles could be unaware of the ways in which some black female dancers could move their hips, buttocks and thighs. I had been a happy witness to this at least since I started attending London's Notting Hill Carnival and West Indian parties in my teens. It is hardly surprising that twerking provoked the backlash it did among so many commentators: the link between dance and sex had never been more obvious.

Now the anti-sex movement could finally take aim from the moral high ground. Object teamed up with black feminist group Imkaan, created an astroturf campaign to censor music videos called *Rewind and Reframe*, and, with help of the ever-supportive *Guardian*, began to insinuate that Cyrus's twerking was not just sexist, but in some way racist too. *Guardian* journalist Hadley Freeman ludicrously complained that Cyrus had 'culturally appropriated' black people by daring to move her buttocks in a certain way, and having apparently worked herself into an angry froth, described the performance as a 'minstrel show'.[59] Under the guise of anti-racism, here was a white 'liberal' journalist doing what racists had done in the Deep South decades earlier: trying to stop black culture from being adopted by white people. In place of an exhortation not to buy 'negro records', the new left had found new language to express their discomfort that white kids were copying the dance moves of black artists.

Freeman's real problem was revealed in the article when she wrote of Cyrus "adding in a racial element while she copied the dance moves of strippers and bellowed her love of drugs". Black people, nudity and drugs: the triumvirate that has upset white conservatives for centuries. She even dared to invoke (or *appropriate*, perhaps) Martin Luther King, ending the article by stating that she 'had a dream':

> I have a dream that female celebrities will one day feel that they don't need to imitate porn actors on magazine covers and in their stage acts. I have a dream that the predominantly white music world will stop reducing black music to grills and bitches and twerking. And I have a dream that stupid songs about seducing "good girls" will be laughed at instead of sent to No 1.

Freeman's dream, of a world free of strippers, porn, drugs, good girls doing bad things and white people doing black things, is hardly a progressive one. She could have found her dream in Selma, Alabama, in 1963, where King made his famous speech. If any article summed up the 21st-century collapse of the left into ugly conservatism, this one did.

If it had appeared alone, Freeman's article might have simply been a one-off piece representing her own views. But it was not: the *Guardian* was in campaign mode. The piece was handily followed and supported a couple of months later by an article from Imkaan's Ikamara Larasi titled "Why must we accept the casual racism in pop videos?"[60], putting the boot in on Miley Cyrus once again, and adding the 'authenticity' of a black voice to Freeman's messy argument (albeit a black voice with close links to Object). And in case we did not get the message, a month later Larasi wrote another *Guardian* piece, "Sexed-up music videos are everyone's problem".[61] Beyond her two attacks on music videos, Larasi was not again seen in the *Guardian*; her work was done.

In addition to Freeman's and Larasi's contributions, the *Guardian* carried a surreal 'news' piece on the story that 73-year-old Christian singer Cliff Richard also disapproved of Cyrus's behaviour, and he "just hopes she grows out of it".[62]

However clumsy and quasi-racist it might have been, the *Guardian*'s attack on 'sexualised music videos' helped do the trick. It was never about convincing Cyrus fans – the goal was to put pressure on the UK authorities. Just one month after Larasi's second article, in January 2014, the *Guardian* wrote in approving terms that the BBFC wanted to regulate (i.e. censor) music videos in the same way it did feature films. Of course it did: the BBFC, let us not forget, is a private business.

> Following the issuing of new classification guidance from the BBFC on Monday, the organisation's assistant director, David Austin, said it was responding to pressure from parents who were concerned about the sexual imagery freely available to children who had access to the web...[63]

And a few months afterwards, in August 2014, the Prime Minister David Cameron announced in a speech on (ominously) The Family that the government was backing censorship of music videos:

> From October, we're going to help parents protect their children from some of the graphic content in online music videos by working with the British Board of Film Classification, Vevo and YouTube to pilot the age rating of these videos.

The Big Panic had claimed an important cultural scalp. Without any genuine public discussion or outcry, and certainly without any research showing that 'sexualised music videos' were causing any harm to anyone, music – and especially black music – would be subject to prurient censorship controls. The old Citizens Council of Greater New Orleans would be proud.

Music companies, who need to reach a teenage audience via

Vevo and YouTube, would have no choice but to self-censor. Just as with porn DVDs, which are often released in a European and a softer UK cut, music videos would be censored for the UK market.

Race and Porn

'Sexualised music videos' provide a good example of how the puritanical ideas of the new left have inevitably led to the adoption of positions that, not so long ago, were more usually associated with the far-right. In recent decades, the demographics of the left have changed sharply. It has become wealthier and whiter, and this has caused deep changes in ideas and attitudes. While it continues to rail loudly against the older, more blatant forms of racism, racist ideas have infected parts of the left; discussion of sex tends to bring these bubbling to the surface.

The 'cultural appropriation' idea visited earlier gives a good example of this. While once, progressives welcomed cultural exchanges and mixing, and the racist right hated these things, now white people are told by left-wingers to leave other people's cultures alone. The reasoning given for this is generally contorted and sometimes funny. Ultimately, the arguments make little sense, which explains why the *Guardian* felt the need to wheel out a black commentator, Ikamara Larasi, to echo its conservative position over censoring music videos. "Look, we have a black friend and she agrees with us!" the coverage screamed.

All this is the result of the left's recent obsession with identity politics. Now, the strength of an argument depends not on what is said, but who says it. A black person is considered to be more authoritative than a white person, on the basis that they are patronisingly deemed to be 'oppressed'. It seems churlish to point out that black people, like white people, have diverse opinions. In order to win such a childish debate, one is forced to find one's own black person to respond: "My black person says your black person is wrong!" We send our token black friends into battle with each other like latter-day gladiators. Just as it has rejected Liberty – at least in the form of free expression – so the left-wing counter-Enlightenment also scorns Reason and Equality. The joining of hands between far-right and new left appears to be complete; the circle is joined.

One of the most overtly racist articles I can remember reading in a mainstream publication in recent years was written in 2009 by the broadcaster Tim Samuels, and published in the *Guardian's* online Comment is Free section. The article promoted Hardcore Profits, a series Samuels had made for the BBC about pornography, for which he visited Ghana in West Africa. As with Hadley Freeman's twerking-induced horror, Samuels has a clear anti-porn agenda, and is so keen to push it that he forgets not to be racist.

Formulaically, Samuels begins his porn condemnation with a disclaimer to show how pro-sex and down-with-the-kids he really is:

> I used to think porn was tremendously good fun. The adolescent thrill of sneaking a copy of Fiesta home inside the Manchester Evening News. Crowding around a PC at university as a smutty picture revealed itself pixel by pixel. Even the equine VHS shown during my first job at GQ gave everyone a good, if not queasy, lads-mag laugh.[64]

He is apparently unaware that, by the time of writing his article, the bestiality material he admits having a laugh over was criminalised as extreme porn, and could now have earned him a prison sentence under Section 63 of the Criminal Justice and Immigration Act 2008.

He then proceeds to explain that porn is not as cool as he thought. Why? Because now, Africans are watching it!

The moment porn truly stopped being fun came in a remote Ghanaian village – mud huts, barefoot kids, no electricity... One of the unforeseen consequences of globalisation is the shocking effect that western porn is having in parts of the developing world.

What is this 'shocking effect'?

The village has no electricity, but that doesn't stop a generator from being wheeled in, turning a mud hut into an impromptu porn cinema – and turning some young men into rapists...

Why does porn turn Ghanaian men into rapists, but not Tim and his mates? This is not spelled out. But clearly these barefoot young men are made of something altogether different from upstanding young British men. There is no statistical evidence provided to show that access to porn correlates with a rise in sexual violence in Ghana, but Samuels instead presents anecdotal evidence from villagers. The statistics from Europe and America (to be examined later) suggest the reverse effect: sexual violence falls as porn availability increases. One might expect the same correlation to take place in Africa: but not if one believes that Africans are somehow different to Westerners.

Samuels links other bad things in African society to porn. HIV, for example: "other young men are buying bootlegs copies [sic] of the almost always condom-free LA-made porn – copying directly what they see and contracting HIV". Copying directly! Those lovable, childlike Africans think that if bareback sex is good enough for the white man, it's good enough for them! HIV has, of course, been rife in Africa since long before DVD players or the Internet have been available. The good news is that its prevalence is declining: in fact, the UN was already reporting a decline in new infections globally[65] even before Samuels blessed Ghana with his enlightened presence. So in fact, it appears that global porn access correlates with a *decline* in HIV. I would not, of course, claim a causal relationship here, but Samuels is, although the statistics appear to contradict him.

Here is a Victorian viewpoint updated for the 21st century. Samuels walks in the footsteps of colonial-era missionaries who strived to encourage African women to cover their nakedness, convert to Christianity and reject polygamy. He indicates a desire to stop all this rape and unsafe sex – which he seems to think is a particularly African problem – and like Gail Dines, blames porn, and inflates the size and power of the porn industry. "Surely this multibillion-dollar industry needs to take some responsibility for the human costs?" Like the colonialists of old, he merely seeks to protect Africans from themselves. And although he seems convinced that these human costs are very real, he does not quantify them, nor explain what the porn industry is supposed to do to clear up its alleged mess. Perhaps each scene could open with a health warning made especially for brown people, explaining that condoms are good, and rape is bad, and African men should do as the white man says, not as he does.

'Sexist' Advertising

Moral panics about advertising are nothing new. In 1957, it was announced that an experiment with subliminal adverts – messages flashed too quickly during a film for the conscious mind to acknowledge – had been shown to influence people's choice of product. This caused a panic at the time over the potential for mind control, but it proved to be untrue. More recently, some studies in subliminal advertising, in very controlled conditions, have shown limited results in improving brand awareness, but the idea that such techniques could fundamentally change people's behaviour appears to be mythical. But there is something about us that enjoys being scared by conspiracy theories about powerful people trying to control us.

While we might not be susceptible to subliminal advertising, we all enjoy a good panic: none of us is immune to a scary story pitched in the right way.

As 'anti-capitalism' has become fashionable – an indication of the left's nihilistic switch in emphasis from building a new system to merely smashing the old one – so we become ever easier to convince that evil corporations are doing unspeakable things for profit; and for sure, there are countless true stories of corporate bad behaviour that make these anti-corporate myths easy to believe. As I write this, my Facebook friends are sharing countless myths about poisons in food and drink, 'chemtrails' that deliberately poison our air, the 'dangers' of fluoride in water, genetically modified 'frankenfoods', 'dangerous' vaccines, 'natural remedies' suppressed by 'big pharma' and on and on.

The idea that capitalism deliberately tries to change us for its own evil purposes has already been encountered in this book: Gail Dines and other anti-pornography campaigners claim that the purpose of the porn industry is not (just) to make money, but – like a cluster of evil scientists – to actually change human sexuality. The Patriarchy, for reasons that are never quite made clear, is determined to turn us all into perverts.

Similarly, advertising aimed at women, and advertising featuring attractive women, is portrayed by activists as 'sexist', and presented as proof that male-dominated capitalism seeks to 'create body-image issues' in women for a variety of vaguely explained but scary-sounding reasons. This does not explain why capitalism does not do the same to men. After all, capitalism seeks nothing more than profit. And certainly, businesses will happily sell unnecessary products to men whenever they get the chance. Ludicrously expensive watches, sports equipment, technical gadgets and – yes – pornography are primarily bought by men.

In truth, men and women are interested (whether for reasons of nature or nurture) in buying different things, and capitalism simply does not work in the way that the conspiracy theorists suggest. To market products towards people that do not want them is expensive, and fundamentally bad for business. Marketeers follow demand; to try to *create* demand is almost certainly doomed to fail. It is only in the rarest cases that a new product – the smartphone comes to mind as a recent example – creates a new market.

But the anti-sex movement is constantly in a state of seething rage about sexist advertising ('sexist' having been redefined for the purposes of the Big Panic to mean 'sexual'), and determined to put an end to it. To make life easier for morality campaigners, British advertising is censored in a similar way to television. The Advertising Standards Authority says its mandate is to prevent advertising that is "misleading, harmful or offensive".[66] While the avoidance of misleading adverts may be a commendable goal, harm (as we have seen) means whatever censors want it to mean, and offensiveness is entirely subjective. This means the ASA has a near-infinite mandate to censor anything, so long as somebody complains about it. As with TV, advertising censorship works in response to small numbers of complaints from 'members of the public', and a handful of complaints by activists can result in an advert being banned.

Predictably, Object and other pro-censorship groups seized the opportunity to censor advertising containing imagery that offended their Victorian sensibilities. A Facebook declaration that an ad was sexist would easily generate enough complaints from Object supporters for the ASA to investigate.

One of the worst examples of this censorship in action was a YouTube commercial for the Renault Clio, which received just a single complaint, and was banned by the ASA in 2013 on the basis that it was harmful/offensive because it "objectified women". The ruling needs to be seen in its entirety to appreciate its moralistic nature. One could imagine similar language coming from a Ministry of Feminine Purity in a dystopian, Orwellian future:

Ad

A YouTube ad for a car, entitled "Two Unsuspecting Guys Take the Renault Clio for a Test Drive" featured hidden camera footage of two men taking a car for a test drive around London. They reached a junction and pressed a button on the dashboard which read "Va Va Voom". A screen, which featured a Parisian scene, was moved into position in front of the car and a number of actors and props appeared, including a man on a scooter, a couple at a café table and a market stall. A group of women then walked in front of the car, wearing burlesque style lingerie and danced in a line in front of the car before walking towards it and gyrating and dancing around it. One woman blew a kiss to the driver. The women then walked away in unison and the screen was moved away to reveal a billboard poster which read "Reignite your Va Va Voom".

Issue

The complainant challenged whether the ad was offensive, because she felt it objectified women.

Response

Renault UK Ltd (Renault) said the video had only been made available on YouTube and was generally intended to be viewed by a younger adult audience than mainstream TV channels. They said the video was a humorous parody with a theme of French culture and it therefore featured various iconic scenes that were associated with Paris, including the Eiffel Tower and a pavement cafe. They said the women who danced around the vehicle were a reference to the Moulin Rouge and that they were intended to be taken as seriously as the other iconic images in the ad. They felt they were dressed in typical Parisian style and that the choreography was a rhythmical send up of the burlesque style, rather than overtly sexual. They advised that the video had been viewed over three million times and they were unaware of any other complaints.

YouTube said the ad did not violate their Community Guidelines or Advertising Policies, but that it was the advertiser's responsibility to ensure that any ad complied with the CAP Code and was targeted appropriately.

Assessment

Upheld

The ASA noted that Renault felt the female dancers were just one of the iconic Parisian scenes featured in the ad, which was intended to be a light-hearted parody. However, we considered that the length of the scene in question, along with the change in the music and the use of slow motion shots, meant it had a different tone to the rest of the ad. We accepted that the Moulin Rouge was associated with Paris and that a scene that referenced it could therefore have some relevance to the theme of the ad, if not to the product itself. However, we were concerned that the ad featured a number of shots of the women's breasts and bottoms, in which their heads were obscured, and which we considered invited viewers to view the women as sexual objects. We further considered that the choreography, dress and facial expressions of the dancers were sexually provocative and that the overall impression given was not necessarily that of a parody of a cabaret show such as the Moulin Rouge, particularly as the women were seen to approach the car and gyrate around it, rather than merely performing in front of it. We considered that the ad objectified the dancers by portraying them as sexual objects and that it was therefore likely to cause serious or widespread offence.

The ad breached CAP Code (Edition 12) rule 4.1 (Harm and offence).

Action

The ad must not appear again in its current form.[67]

As if to underline the sexist nature of this ruling, Renault had produced two similar versions of the ad: one featuring women, and one showing 'objectified' men. Even the *Daily Mail* noticed the hypocrisy:

> Intriguingly, an almost exact mirror-image version of the same advert – this time featuring a woman driver surrounded by a group of hunky, scantily clad, bare-chested and gyrating men as if in a scene from the Full Monty – received nearly a million online 'hits' but no complaints and is therefore free to continue to be aired unchanged, the ASA confirmed.[68]

Orwell fans might recognise the doublethink here. The right of women to appear as unashamedly sexual beings was being attacked by an unelected bureaucracy in the name of 'combatting sexism'. In *1984*, the English Socialist Society had a slogan: War is Peace; Freedom is Slavery; Ignorance is Strength. To this, we might add: Oppression is Liberation.

But this power to censor-by-complaint was not enough for the moral entrepreneurs. Object began a campaign for 'sexist' ads to be made illegal across the European Union, with a petition at change.org stating:

> The media have a great responsibility in promoting equality between women and men. For too long, the representations of women have been misused by the media advertising; we continue, as people working for equality, to fight against stereotypes. More and more often and louder, we say NO to sexist advertising![69]

Women's Rights: Not For All Women

One of the ironies of opposing sexual expression from a feminist standpoint is that most of the money to be earned from it is earned by women. Not only is there far more work for women in pornography, modelling and striptease, but women in these fields are far better paid than men. Despite popular mythology (much of it created by anti-sex campaigners) that depicts sex-related work as male-run and exploitative, the business of sex has mostly been dominated and run by women throughout its history. Anti-sex feminists tend to say "women shouldn't have to earn money from sex", but this is a straw-man argument: nobody is suggesting this, and women do not *have* to earn money from sex: but they can, if they choose. The anti-sex message is really: "women shouldn't earn money from sex under any circumstances".

Various female friends and acquaintances that I have met during my work in the porn industry and my sexual-freedom activism have created for themselves lifestyles of which many men would be envious – myself included. There is the friend who funded years of world travel by working as a stripper, and never having to do any work she did not enjoy. The woman who spent several years travelling, partying and selling sex from time to time when the cash ran out. The 23-year-old graduate who moved to London and earns a six-figure income as a sex worker, and whose 'business plan' involves becoming mistress to a rich man who will buy her a flat. The pornstar who paid her way through university. The pornstar who owned a London flat, before retiring in her early 30s to start a family. The various pornstars who can afford to spend months at a time partying in Ibiza or Thailand. The older women who worked in the phone-sex business in the 1990s, and their younger equivalents who do webcam work today, for whom 'going to work' means putting on some make-up and switching on their PC.

The downside for all these women is that the work usually has to come to an end. Few that I have met in these industries intend to keep doing sex-related work beyond 40 (though there are exceptions). I have seen the sadness of strippers and pornstars who have to quit the job they loved for something they often do not: the horror of the 'nine to five' haunts them. But this is the downside of having choice, not (as some try to claim) of coercion.

In the past, feminism was not about closing down female choice, but making new choices available: enabling those women who wanted to become plumbers, business managers or pilots but not disempowering those who wanted to be glamour models, mistresses or sex workers. Anti-sex feminism is ironic therefore, because it tries to destroy the lifestyles that are, and have always been, female-dominated, as well as lucrative.

When women's rights are invoked by anti-sex feminists, they are referring to a narrow set of rights that many people would see as bogus: the right to walk into a supermarket without seeing a bikini-clad model on the cover of a lads' mag. The right to sit on the train without the risk of getting a glimpse of Page 3. The right to *not* see attractive female bodies in advertising. These dubious rights are created to undermine other, genuine rights for other women: the right to work; the right to self-expression; the right to dress, undress and present one's own body as one chooses; the right to define one's own sexuality.

Rights are complex and can conflict with each other: a right to religious freedom does not extend to carrying out human sacrifice, for example, because one person's right to life overrides another's right to practise their religion. But anti-sex feminists not only claim that their rights are infringed by the choices of other women, but their rights *override* those of other women. The woman who feels threatened by the existence of Page 3 has stronger rights (she thinks) than the woman who is paid to model for Page 3. In this world-view, the right to moral outrage trumps the right to work. This is an abuse of the concept of human rights.

The clever use of porn-panic words – in particular 'objectification' – helps to support this twisted reasoning. To say "I am objectified by that model's choice to pose naked because she and I are both women" is nonsensical, but that does not stop people from saying it. This thinking has leaked from the morality movement into mainstream discourse. I have often been invited to discuss in media interviews and university debates whether

"Porn objectifies or empowers [all] women". The answer is neither: unless you have personally appeared in a porn scene, you have been neither empowered nor objectified by it. By trying to claim that another woman's choices have objectified *you*, you are merely finding an excuse to control *her*. This attempt to claim that one woman's choices can affect *all* women is fundamentally authoritarian, providing a blueprint for anybody to attack the rights of others on the flimsiest grounds. This tribal thinking is an inevitable outcome of the identity politics that has become so fashionable in the past decade.

The Great November Panic

As the Big Panic matured, new claims about the dangers of free expression appeared more and more frequently, and opposition became muted. The purpose of moral panic is to make the extreme seem normal, and previously acceptable ideas seem extreme.

A storm of panic was driven by the old-fashioned conservative belief that women, once again the weaker sex, were in need of special protection from things that might offend or (in unexplained ways) harm them. Moral entrepreneurs also became better at selecting unsympathetic targets and generating social-media storms against them.

Three moral panics that all surfaced in November 2014 illustrated the pro-censorship zeitgeist: Dapper Laughs, Julien Blanc and Shirtgate.

Stand-up comedian Daniel O'Reilly, better known as his laddish character Dapper Laughs, had built a large online following and been given his own show on ITV2, which attracted claims of sexism. When a video appeared of O'Reilly (in character as Dapper) at a live show, telling a female audience member she was "gagging for a rape", the inevitable social-media eruption followed. Like most of his critics, I had not heard of Dapper Laughs until the panic broke: the video clip looked ugly, but to draw an opinion of a comedy character based on a few seconds of out-of-context video seemed kneejerk in the extreme. When the inevitable petition attracted over 68,000 signatures, O'Reilly's TV show was cancelled by ITV, as was his live tour. He had been branded 'sexist', 'misogynist' and a contributor to 'rape culture' by people who, by and large, had never seen his show.

I was informed by various feminist acquaintances that Dapper Laughs was 'vile'; like Mary Whitehouse in her heyday, many of his fiercest attackers happily admitted to have not seen any of the material they were denouncing. One female friend who, rather than follow the crowd, decided to make up her own mind, sought out some of his videos online, and told me she found them funny rather than offensive. When I examined tweets directed at Dapper Laughs after the cancellation of his show, many came from female fans who expressed upset and bemusement that the programme was no longer to be broadcast. Why would someone so horribly misogynistic have a strong female following? No doubt, a 'feminist analysis' would suggest his female fans had been 'steeped in a culture of misogyny' which had led them to hate their own gender and find O'Reilly amusing, but this reasoning is unlikely, and merely attempts to intellectualise the basest witch-hunting behaviour. The definition of 'censor' as one who supervises the manners or morality of others seemed to fit perfectly. As in so many similar cases of moral panic, there were signs of class war around the whole affair. Those who wished to enjoy his comedy had been censored by those, more socially powerful, who did not want *anyone* to see it. In Cultural-Revolution style, O'Reilly was dragged through TV studios to apologise for himself, though his fans had never asked him to.

The second November panic arose over an American 'pick-up artist', Julien Blanc, who had planned a trip to the UK to run seminars on how to attract women. Blanc's promotional videos implied that he was teaching men how to 'trick' women into being attracted to them, and this was again seized upon as the promotion of 'rape culture'. Blanc's marketing messages were perhaps clumsy and ill-advised, and his presentation crudely laddish, but the panic was overblown, as panics are: no law had been broken, no victims had been found.

Once Blanc's name had been associated with that vague-yet-frightening thing 'rape culture', the bandwagon began rolling again. This time, the petition (calling on the Home Secretary to deny Blanc an entry visa) exceeded 150,000 signatures. Conservative and Labour MPs united to express their horror, and the minister duly barred Blanc from entering the country. A chilling statement proudly boasted that: "This home secretary has excluded more foreign nationals on the grounds of unacceptable behaviour than any before her".

Commentators of the left, usually wary of heavy-handed restrictions on immigration, instead applauded the decision. To illustrate that the panic was international, Australia took similar action against Blanc, with its right-wing immigration minister saying: "This guy wasn't putting forward political ideas. He was putting forward abuse that was derogatory to women and those values are abhorred in this country."[70] Any form of expression that anyone might describe as sexist now appeared to be fair game for the witch-hunters. This Australian example illustrates how the rhetoric of anti-sexism, once used by the left to fight for women's rights, had now also been adopted by the right in order to justify authoritarianism, as well as to subtly imply that women can no longer handle being treated as equal to men.

Next in line was Matt Taylor, a scientist involved with the Rosetta project, which landed a space probe on a faraway comet. This was one of mankind's greatest ever scientific achievements. As if to illustrate the anti-intellectualism of the pro-censorship movement, a few people were more concerned with the fact that Taylor wore a handmade shirt at a press conference, than with humanity's latest step forward. The shirt's material displayed sexual (or 'sexist', in the eyes of morality campaigners) cartoon pictures of women, and the Big Panic, triumphant in its recent humbling of O'Reilly and Blanc, prepared to take its third scalp.

However, this time, the attack was ill-chosen. Forced to apologise on TV, with his supportive team sitting by, and now wearing a drab hoodie, Taylor burst into tears. The greatest moment of his life had become one of his worst. Public support for him rallied. The moralists were forced even further onto the back foot when it emerged that the shirt had been made by a female artist friend of Taylor's, who came forward to express puzzlement that her art might be considered sexist. For a moment, the crusaders were exposed as authoritarian bullies.

The backfiring of Shirtgate created a temporary pause in the Big Panic, and revealed a basic truth. Most people appeared to have no objection to the kinds of expression that were now being presented as sexist. The panic was driven by small, well-organised groups that had become adept at whipping up moral outrage in regular bursts. Online petitions take seconds to sign. Even 150,000 people signing a petition represented less than a quarter of one percent of the UK population. One person making a complaint to Ofcom or the ASA represented nobody but themselves.

The authoritarian, bullying climate was noticed by an older generation of feminists. Of all the journalists who might flag up the problem of what I call the Big Panic, Julie Bindel was one I would have least expected to intervene. Bindel, a veteran radical feminist, and vociferous anti-porn and anti-prostitution campaigner, may not have been considered a natural friend of free expression, especially of the 'lad culture' variety, but she turned on those who had attacked Dapper Laughs, Julien Blanc and Matt Taylor, blaming them for doing damage to the feminist movement. In a *Guardian* piece with the title "Feminism is in danger of becoming toxic", she wrote:

The current climate of McCarthyism within some segments of feminism and the left is so ingrained and toxic that there are active attempts to outlaw some views because they cause offence. Petitions against individuals appear to be a recent substitute for political action towards the root causes of misogyny and other social ills. Petitions have taken over politics.[71]

Tyler, The Creator

Possibly, Britain's Home Secretary Theresa May had been gratified by the acclaim she had received for banning Julien Blanc from Britain. This episode provided a valuable lesson for right-wing authoritarians like May: so long as acts of censorship are dressed up in the right language, nobody with any clout will oppose them.

The next ban of an 'unsuitable foreigner' was a breathtakingly pointless piece of cultural (and probably racial) bullying. Tyler, The Creator, a young, black American hip-hop artist, was barred from the UK (where he had been planning to tour) in August 2015. The basis of the ban was that he had written and performed misogynistic and homophobic lyrics several years earlier, at the age of 18. There could have been no serious suggestion that Tyler was any kind of threat to anyone – especially since his lyrics were no longer of the crude kind that had once caused offence. But now, his mere physical presence was deemed to be a significant enough problem that he should be barred from entering the country.

The smell of witch-hunt was again in the air. Some primitive human fear instinct had elevated a young man who had once penned some unpleasant words to the status of kryptonite; merely being in his presence might turn young British men into violent rapists and homophobes! The 'rape culture' meme came into play. While rape is measurable, rape culture is not. It is the superstitious idea that rape somehow hangs in the air and infects people like a virus. Carriers must be quarantined.

The hand of pro-censorship feminism was again visible. Collective Shout, an Australian feminist group with a history of anti-porn campaigning, had already successfully petitioned to have Tyler banned from Australia based on his lyrics and alleged bad behaviour. The British ban merely rubber-stamped the earlier Australian decision. Where have all the racists gone? Leftward. They appear to have realised that lynching a black man is no longer OK; unless you first label him a misogynist. Then it's fine.

Hip hop has long been a proxy for racism. It is a black art-form that has lasted decades and grown from strength to strength. Although a creation of New York City, it encapsulates the African excellence in rhythmic, spoken-word performance. It has elevated poetry to new heights and become the world's most widely adopted musical form, in every language. It is common to hear hip hop dismissed in its entirety as 'cRap' (geddit?). This makes no more sense than to dismiss all poetry, or all guitar music. Hip hop infuriates because it represents a global triumph of something uniquely African.

Small, forgettable events like the inexplicable travel ban on a young American man are litmus tests for our political system and societal attitudes. Our culture does not appear to be in a good place right now.

Revolution!

Amidst the authoritarian and censorious attitudes, talk of revolution was in the air. Perhaps the younger generation was noticing that the social revolutions of the 1960s were imperilled, and was ready to mount a defence! But perhaps not.

This revolution was led by comedian and self-styled Messiah figure Russell Brand. Brand's style of comedy was verbally playful, super-energetic, rambling, surreal and very funny, and he had attracted a large fan base. His earlier heroin addiction and outrageous sexual exploits only endeared Brand more to his fans.

But he had never been a satirist, nor shown any great interest in politics before. His boundless energy, unleashed as he looked for ways to turn away from his compulsive behaviours towards drugs and sex, was directed instead into political campaigning.

The combination of charisma, a ready-made following, media presence, idealism and energy can be dangerous when coupled with a trusting nature and political naivety. Brand was a populist who appeared to absorb ideas like a sponge from those around him. His message was a nihilistic one, and anti-democratic. Like so many revolutionaries before him, Brand wanted to smash rather than fix, and to preach rather than learn. His call to boycott the ballot box appealed to the apolitical: it takes far less effort to say "They're all the same, I'm not voting" than try to understand where one's vote is best directed. Nigel Farage, leader of the right-wing and nationalistic UKIP, may have been attention-seeking when he said he and Brand were "not so different, you and I"[72], but he was not completely wrong either: both were playing on apathy and disillusion by presenting British democracy as beyond repair. As if to demonstrate his confusion, Brand reversed his stance over boycotting the ballot box days before the election, but too late for many people (including, presumably, himself) to register to vote.

Brand surrounded himself with voices of the new left, and so inevitably absorbed their puritanism. Like many reformed addicts, he seemed to feel that his compulsive behaviours gave him a special insight into the human condition, and so he had the right to stop other people going down the same paths, even if, unlike Brand, they possessed some degree of self-control. So it was of little surprise when he turned his revolutionary zeal against sexual expression, pontificating in language that could just as easily have come from a Christian fundamentalist:

Our attitudes towards sex have become warped and perverted and have deviated from its true function as an expression of love and a means for procreation... there's just icebergs of filth floating through every house on Wi-Fi... It's inconceivable what it must be like to be an adolescent boy now with this kind of access to porn. It must be dizzying and exciting, yet corrupting in a way we can't even imagine.[73]

We learn that sex has 'true' functions, and 'fun' is not among them.

Revolutionaries, like censors, are elitists who feel they have a special right to control the lives and destinies of others. Many revolutions, created in blind idealism, end up creating a path to power for people even worse than the old, toppled elite. The anarchist feminist Emma Goldman knew this when she said of puritanical revolutionaries who would sacrifice all humanity for The Cause: "If I can't dance, I don't want your revolution!"

Addiction to Porn

The Big Panic had united a wide array of people around the idea that free expression had gone too far. Across the political spectrum and the mass media, from feminists to religious fundamentalists, from the girl guides to Russell Brand: the pus-filled boil of pro-censorship fear and loathing was swollen and ready to burst.

Those of us who had been watching carefully knew that website-blocking had long been on the agenda; we did not know when or how it would be introduced. We could, however, guess that pornography would figure in the justification. I began writing this book on the assumption that Internet freedom in the UK would fundamentally come under attack while I was writing; and was proven right.

The beginning of the end was signalled, in late-March 2015, by a press release from the National Society for the Prevention of Cruelty to Children (NSPCC), which had carried out a study into the impacts of pornography on young people. Or that was how it was headlined: what they had actually done was commission an online poll by a PR company called OnePoll.

OnePoll does not carry out research that would hold any weight in academia. The company carries out the kind of fluff 'research' that all too often appears in newspapers in place of real news, and helps plug products on behalf of OnePoll's clients. *Management Today* had previously carried a scathing article on OnePoll and similar PR companies under the headline: "The 'research' that isn't actually research... It's time for the PR industry to clean up its act."[74]

In the case of the NSPCC's porn study, OnePoll had simply sent an 11-question poll out to members of its regular research base (who get paid a small amount for each poll completed), asking them to hand the keyboard to their child to complete the questionnaire. One of the first questions asked was whether the child is addicted to pornography.

This is wrong at several levels: is the child really completing the survey, or is the (paid) parent doing it for them? Is it ethically right to ask a child such a question online, when their parent might be watching their responses? Does it make any sense to ask someone – adult or child – to self-diagnose in this way? But most important, the very existence of porn addiction, although popularised in the mass media, is viewed with a high degree of scepticism by psychologists. Why was the NSPCC asking children if they suffer from an ailment that might not even exist?

Moral panics over some new form of addiction regularly raise their heads. Everything from computer games and mobile phones to sex and porn have been labelled addictive. The NSPCC is a veteran of the panic game, having also participated in the early-80s video-nasties moral panic, submitting research that claimed young children were accessing adult videos. Its trusted brand is doubtless useful in helping make the case for controls on free expression on the basis of 'protecting children'.

The flexible concept of addiction suits many interests: censors who want to label something dangerous in order to justify regulation, newspapers looking for scare stories and therapists with cures to peddle. Addiction also provides a convenient excuse for people who indulge in certain behaviours: the golfer Tiger Woods, having been caught out in a long string of extra-marital affairs and losing valuable sponsors, conveniently discovered he was suffering from 'sex addiction' and checked into rehab, later to emerge 'clean' and ready to resume his lucrative career.

Psychologist and author Dr David Ley, who specialises in this field, is highly critical of those who invoke such addictions:

> Sex and porn can cause problems in people's lives, just like any other human behavior or form of entertainment. But, to invoke the idea of 'addiction' is unethical, using invalid, scientifically and medically-rejected concepts to invoke fear and feed panic.[75]

A psychology study at Case Western University looked at people who believed they were addicted to porn, and found that while the amount of porn-viewing did not affect the levels of 'addiction', religious beliefs did. Those who had been raised with conservative attitudes towards sex were more likely to see their porn-viewing as problematic, and to be distressed by it. The study's author, Dr Joshua Grubbs, noted that whether or not 'porn addiction' could be considered real, *perceived* addiction was a problem that could lead to depression, compulsive behaviour and anxiety.[76] Seen in this light, the NSPCC poll was more than just dodgy research; it was deeply unethical, and likely to amplify teenage anxiety over their own normal sexual responses.

The survey was released to the media with the 'shock' headline that around a tenth of 12 and 13 year olds were worried they might be addicted to pornography, and was widely reported.[77] My first reaction was that, if in response to such provocative questioning, only a tenth of the respondents reported fear of addiction, that seemed like a very low number. In a society less prone to panic, this might even have been reported as good news.

The Tipping Point

The purpose of a moral panic is to create the conditions for an authoritarian response.

Days after the NSPCC had fed the media a tale of porn-addicted children (handily, the NSPCC story was issued during an election campaign), the Tories announced that, should they win the election, they would introduce an official Internet censor for the first time. Naturally, they were not nearly that straight-forward: the announcement was buried in the middle of an extremely long and predictable Facebook rant about pornography. The meat of the announcement was as follows (with my italics):

So today we are announcing that, if the Conservatives win the next General Election, we will legislate to put online hard-core pornography behind effective age verification controls.

Of course adults should be perfectly free to look at these sites. But if websites showing adult content don't have proper age controls in place – ones that will stop children looking at this kind of material – *they should and will be blocked altogether.* No sex shop on the high street would be allowed to remain open if it knowingly sold pornography to underage customers, and there is no reason why the internet should be any different.

An independent regulator will oversee this new system. It will determine, in conjunction with websites, how age verification controls will work and how websites that do not put them in place will be blocked.[78]

While the requirement for age verification looks reasonable at first glance, in practise this announcement had huge implications. As discussed earlier, the age-verification requirement in the AVMS 2014 law made well over 99% of all porn sites (and much, much else besides) illegal in the UK. Millions of sites would be permanently blocked to all UK users under this apparently innocuous policy.

True to form, Labour's response entirely ignored the threat to free expression, and instead tried to paint the Tories as not-tough-enough, with Chris Bryant saying:

> After five years of inaction by the Tories, this proposal is too little too late. Protecting children from inappropriate material both on and offline should be a priority but the Tories have failed to act quickly enough.[79]

But all of this ignored a key point: amidst the rising atmosphere of panic, nobody had produced a smoking gun. If porn was causing harm, where was the evidence?

8

Porn: What's the Harm?

Make the lie big, make it simple, keep saying it, and eventually they will believe it – Adolf Hitler

The seeds of the porn panic, which has blossomed in Britain and internationally over the past decade, were sown in the United States almost half a century ago, when the Supreme Court decided that pornography was protected expression under the First Amendment. A decade later, Dworkin and MacKinnon crafted much of the language that is still deployed against pornography today, and laid the groundwork for social conservatives to begin their long journey from right to left of the political spectrum.

One might expect that after so many years, the campaigns against pornography, strip clubs, sex work and sexualised-everything would have assembled an armory of evidence to back their positions. After all, if one sought evidence that sexual expression was in some way harmful, where better to find it than from the anti-sex movement, which has been making claims of harm for decades?

But quite simply, anti-porn advocates are at a loss when asked to present hard evidence that pornography – or any form of sexual expression – is harmful. The fact that the anti-porn movement cannot provide compelling research or statistical evidence to back its case, and instead relies on moral panic, hyperbole, personal attack and anecdote, should provide a hint as to the true nature of the debate. One can scour anti-porn websites and read Gail Dines books for hours or days without finding a hard fact.

What about the Workers?

I have met a variety of campaigners in debate, with the same sets of stories to tell. Besides the endless repetition of porn-panic mantras, there are usually horrific anecdotes of terrible things done to women within the industry. These generally refer to anonymous ex-performers who the campaigners have rescued (thus justifying the generous grants they receive from worthy organisations). These stories have escalated over the years, as if there is a secret competition to test the public's credulity. In one recent university debate, my opponent was a lawyer who claimed she was involved in rescuing pornstars from abuse. She told of a young woman who had approached her for help, with "green pus leaking out of her vagina".

This produced the desired response of horror from the students, but led me to question why a pornstar with so serious an infection would approach a lawyer rather than a doctor. To anyone familiar with the industry, the story was clearly invented. Nobody is forced to pay greater attention to their sexual health than pornstars. Performers are required to bring STI certificates to each shoot, dated within the past four weeks (or even less, in the case of some studios), and will not be allowed to work if they do not have one. This means that they are tested far more frequently than pretty much anybody else. The industry has developed various health systems to make the testing process as easy as possible, including online lookup services to validate certificates. In Britain, the NHS is aware of pornstars and other sex workers, and provides free, unlimited STI tests. At the slightest hint of an HIV outbreak, the industry shuts down entirely.

Privately, I asked the lawyer whether she had any actual cases I could read about. Any that had resulted in arrests or had reached court would be in the public domain. She could provide none. Here was a rare lawyer who was shy to trumpet her own victories; or more likely, she had never actually encountered a real pornstar in distress.

While there are small numbers of ex-pornstars who campaign against the industry, most have a book to sell, or have found Jesus (Shelley Lubben appears to have cornered this market). And for every one of these, there are countless pornstars who are proud to stand up for their work.

Numerous studies contest the idea that porn work is bad for women: in one 2012 study, published in the *Journal of Sex Research*, the attitudes of 177 female performers were matched against women of similar ages, marital status and other factors. It was found that the pornstars had higher self-esteem and better body images than the average, that they slept better and enjoyed sex more in their private lives.[80] This matches with my own discussions with pornstars, including my friends, who typically enjoy their work and the lifestyle that goes with it, and invariably say that their self-confidence improves when they start porn work. In fact, in my experience, it is usually men that find the work more physically demanding and less enjoyable (for some obvious reasons). Men also feature less prominently than women, and are often used as 'stunt dicks', largely kept off-camera, which instead focuses on the female face and body (some directors, like Anna Span, have tried to remedy this, with greater focus on the male personality). Male performers tend to be paid far less than female ones, and have fewer fans.

Attitude studies among porn users have also failed to match the claims of the anti-porn movement. In fact, such studies appear to show broadly beneficial outcomes: porn users tend to have more progressive attitudes than non-users towards anything from women being in positions of power to gay marriage. These studies do not prove that porn changes attitudes though: it may be that more religious people, holding more conservative attitudes, are also less likely to look at porn. But whatever the explanation, the smoking gun fails to appear. Porn-viewing does not, it seems, lead towards misogyny or other unpleasant attitudes.

The weakness of anti-porn arguments should be good news for campaigners against censorship, but heated public debates are never about reason and careful deliberation. The very purpose of moral panic is to stifle debate and turn truth-telling into heresy. Besides, the goal of anti-sex moral panics is not to win the public argument, but to create the conditions for acts of censorship to take place.

The pornography debate takes a similar form to the climate-change one, with a weight of evidence on one side stacked against well-funded propaganda machines on the other. While decades of serious research have failed to find evidence against porn, the anti-sex movement has been working overtime, establishing porn-panic words and ideas – objectification, sexualisation, porn addiction and so on – into the public consciousness. As already outlined, the movement has proved itself flexible and dynamic, abandoning an overtly religious presentation for a pseudo-liberal one when that became more convincing.

The vested interest of the supposedly mighty and powerful porn industry is juxtaposed against poorly funded campaigners, who valiantly battle against rape and child abuse. But valuations of the porn industry, as presented by the likes of Gail Dines, are vastly exaggerated. More importantly, many porn-industry players – especially the larger companies – see censorship as a remedy to the blight of free content which undermines their profits, and so are on the same side as the anti-porn activists who claim to be working against them. Furthermore, grants and donations are available in abundance to the right kinds of campaigning organisations, and so prohibitionist groups like Object, by labelling themselves women's rights or anti-rape organisations, can win grants. Wealthy religious groups funnel money into the anti-porn crusade. Government regulators require the acceptance of censorship for their very existence. And these forces are joined by the might of global entertainment corporations, which see porn panic as a useful lever with which to introduce blocking of sites encouraging content piracy.

The panic has done its work. When I appear in a radio studio or public debate and make the point that evidence of harm is scarce-to-nonexistent, I have to battle groans from the audience or "Oh come on...!" from the presenter. To quote Orwell again: "In a time of universal deceit – telling the truth is a revolutionary act".

Think Of The Children!

The anti-porn lobby's failure to produce hard evidence for their case is brushed under the carpet. Once put on the spot, its entire argument reduces to: "OK, we can't prove that porn makes people do bad things but *do we really want our children to be seeing this filth?*" Think Of The Children is, of course the ultimate fallback for the person who has lost the argument on every other front. It is, indeed, a hard point to counter, especially when given 20 seconds to do so on Radio 4. However solid one's position might be, to argue against censorship can be presented as a short step away from supporting child abuse.

The presentation of Think Of The Children varies depending on the forum. The anti-porn speaker, faced with the obvious fact that the vast majority of people who watch porn *don't* turn into sexual abusers, will respond along the lines "...of course, there is no *direct* link between watching porn and committing rape... but surely nobody can question the effects on the young mind... objectification... addiction... misogyny... rape culture..."

The media regulator Ofcom more soberly accepts the lack of evidence of harm (including to teenagers), but then invokes the need for a "precautionary approach". The precautionary approach is the closest possible thing to an open admission of deceit, and would not be an acceptable argument in any other forum. In most cases where harm is alleged, the onus is on the accuser to make the case for action. So mandatory seatbelts in cars, and public smoking bans, were introduced only once it was clear beyond doubt that lives would be saved. To muddy the waters, Ofcom instead refers to 'moral harm'; however this is not harm at all, but an admission that its opposition to pornography is driven by moral judgements about sex.

Ofcom's own findings, which are based on research conducted by governments across Europe, were published in an official report produced for the UK government in 2011:

> There seems to be no relationship between the availability of pornography and an increase in sex crimes in other [European] countries; *in comparison there is more evidence for the opposite effect...*
>
> Research with adults indicates no relationship between the commission of sex crimes and use of pornography at an early age. *Again in comparison there is evidence for the opposite effect.*[81] [My italicisation]

The astonishing fact is, therefore, that as far as anyone can tell, porn appears to be broadly beneficial to society – or at least correlates consistently with beneficial outcomes. Not only does porn not turn young men into rapists, but research by European governments suggests it reduces sex crimes. No wonder the pro-censorship lobby is so determined to close down this discussion.

And it is not just Ofcom. The failure to link porn with harm goes all the way back to the US Presidential Commission of the 1960s. The UK's own in-depth study, conducted in the 70s by the Williams Committee, also came to the conclusion that porn was not harmful. These studies have since been replicated worldwide, which explains the lack of urgency in most countries to follow Britain's censorship lead. Most of Europe does not experience the same level of panic over sexual expression, and America (which often does) is constrained from censorship by the First Amendment. Only a handful of democratic nations show similar enthusiasm for censorship: perhaps Ireland, Iceland, Australia and Canada may follow our lead if Britain censors the Internet.

What If We Could Run a Huge Experiment?

In its reports, while admitting it cannot find harm, Ofcom makes the point that it would be unethical to subject minors to pornography in order to study its effects. This is of course true. But it would be useful if millions of people – adults and teenagers across a wide variety of cultures – could be studied after exposure to pornography.

But of course, we *can* do this, and Ofcom takes care in its report to avoid stating the obvious. Not just millions, but hundreds of millions of people of all ages have watched pornography in the past half-century, and access has become increasingly easy during that time. We can therefore try to measure the effects of all this objectification, sexualisation and pornification using statistical techniques. If there are negative effects, as claimed by the pro-censorship lobby, we should be able to measure them.

We can also compare different societies with each other. We know that Denmark was the first country to remove all censorship of pornography, so (assuming porn causes harm) we would expect to find particularly acute problems there.

The United States is a useful source of data, since it comprises 50 states, each somewhat different from the other with regard to wealth, demographics, culture, access to technology and religious attitudes, but all governed by a single system of federal law, and subject to standardised data collection. By comparing states with each other, useful information might appear.

The Mass Effects of Sexualisation and Objectification

If I were a typical member of the anti-porn movement, I would believe that young people are becoming sexualised by everything from advertising and music videos to Page 3 and pornography.

But how to demonstrate this? One obvious metric could be a rise in teenage pregnancies.

In 2015, the Office for National Statistics announced that pregnancies (including those terminated by abortion) among girls under 18 in England and Wales were at their lowest since records began in 1969. The figures showed a startling drop of 13% for girls under 18, between 2012 and 2013, and a 14% drop for girls under 16. According to the *Guardian*, the ONS believed that:

> the drop in the number of underage pregnancies could be explained by several factors, including the improved programmes of sex and relationship education introduced by successive governments.
>
> The report also stated that it could be due to a "shift in aspirations of young women towards education" or the "perception of stigma associated with being a teenage mother".[82]

These explanations seem reasonable. What the coverage failed to note was that these impressive declines coincided with two other phenomena: unprecedented, easy access to free pornography, and a rising moral panic over sexualisation. The *Guardian* notably failed to address the apparent contradiction between its own moralistic coverage of sexualisation and this decline in teenage pregnancy.

I had an opportunity to put this point to a proponent of porn censorship during a radio debate, and was confidently told that the reason for the decline in pregnancy was an increase in the prevalence of anal sex among teenagers caused (of course) by porn. Surveys do indeed seem to show increased sexual adventurousness (quite possibly resulting from porn-viewing), but it seems unlikely that, even if there has been a steep rise in the popularity of anal sex, there would be a huge subsequent decline in vaginal sex. Conversely, there appears to be plenty of anecdotal evidence that anal sex is favoured over vaginal in more conservative societies where female virginity is still prized. This was perhaps best expressed in the Garfunkel and Oates song, *The Loophole*:

Walk the halls of high school with my purity ring
Unlike those other girls, I've got my morals in check
It was easy to do until I got a boyfriend
And pardon my French, but he's cute as heck
But I made a pact
To keep my hymen intact
And Jesus and I are tight
Never learned about the birds and the bees
I was taught to keep an aspirin in between my knees
Cause The Bible says premarital sex is wrong
But Jason says that guys can't wait that long
I don't want to lose him
To someone who'll do him
I need to figure something out
Well there's a loophole in The Scripture that works really well
So I can get him off without going to hell
It's my Hail Mary, full of grace
In Jesus' name we go to fifth base!
Oh, thank you for making me holy
And thank you for giving me holes to choose from
And since I'm not a godless whore
He'll have to come in the back door

Most of the accusations made against pornography are of a vague, subjective nature. The 'objectification' claim loosely suggests that porn leads men and boys to see women and girls as lesser beings, of lower value, whose feelings are therefore discounted. Although this is difficult to measure directly, there must be some measurable modification of mass behaviour as a result of these changed attitudes: in particular one would expect to observe some correlation between porn-viewing and rape. This is, of course, the most consistent and striking claim made against pornography: that it causes men to rape women. If true, it would be far harder to justify an anti-censorship position.

Berl Kutchinsky, professor of Criminology at the University of Copenhagen, made this point in a 1991 paper, *Pornography, Sex Crime and Public Policy*:

> one issue stands out as particularly important: the claim that pornography, or certain forms of pornography, can lead to serious sex crimes, in particular forcible rape. If this can be proved, then there is consensus that pornography, or these particular forms of pornography, should be forbidden. If it cannot be proved that pornography leads to rape, then there is no such consensus. All other forms of alleged harm or offence, such as pornography degrading women, either as models or bystanders, leading to sexual callousness to women, causing moral outrage, encouraging sexual perversion, or causing marital distress, are usually considered too intangible, or unsupported.[83]

Pornography and Rape

Berl Kutchinsky was a researcher into the links between porn and sex crime. Denmark, having been the first country to allow adults uncensored access to pornography, provided useful data on how this freeing of control had affected Danish society. Sweden and West Germany had swiftly followed the Danish lead, and Kutchinsky studied all three countries, along with the more conservative United States.

In the paper quoted above, Kutchinsky compared rates of reported rape in the four countries, over the period from 1964 to 1984. He was studying during an era in which porn, in the form of magazines and then video, had become increasingly widely available. Writing in 1991, he was unaware that a new porn revolution was about to be sparked by the worldwide web.

Kutchinsky's study found that reported rates of sex crime were effectively flat in Germany during the period covered, and saw very slight rises in Denmark and Sweden. Meanwhile in the USA, rates had increased fairly sharply until about 1979, when they had plateaued. He pointed to evidence that the likelihood of reporting rape in Denmark and Sweden increased between 1964 and 1984:

> In both cases it is likely that at least some of the increase is due to increased reporting and registration of rape, as a result of growing awareness of the rape problem among women as well as the police. There are strong indications that even in the USA, the increase of rape since the mid-1970s may be due to increased reporting/registration.

From 1971, Germany began to record more detail about sexual offences, and so Kutchinsky was able to note that the more serious sexual offences were actually declining; and the more serious the offence, the steeper the decline:

> there is a marked decreasing tendency in the two most serious types of rape. In fact, between 1971 and 1987 group rapes decreased 59 per cent from 577 to 239 cases while rape by strangers decreased 33 per cent from 2453 to 1655 cases (this decrease has continued through 1988 and 1989).

So Kutchinsky showed that, in the two decades up to 1984, the rise in availability of pornography did not appear to drive an increase in rape: in fact, the opposite appeared to be happening. The report's conclusion was clear:

> The aggregate data on rape and other violent or sexual offences from four countries where pornography, including

aggressive varieties, has become widely and easily available during the period we have dealt with would seem to exclude, beyond any reasonable doubt, that this availability has had any detrimental effects in the form of increased sexual violence. The data from West Germany is striking since here, the only increase in sexual violence takes place in the form which includes the least serious forms of sexual coercion and where there may have been increases in reporting frequency. As far as the other forms of sexual violence are concerned, the remarkable fact is that they decreased the more so, the more serious the offence.

This finding is not so strange. Most other research data we have about pornography and rape suggest that the link between them is more than weak. Our knowledge about the contents, the uses and the users of pornography suggests that pornography does not represent a blueprint for rape, but is essentially an aphrodisiac, that is, food for the sexual fantasy of persons mostly males who like to masturbate.

However, compared to today, porn was still a rare and difficult-to-access commodity in 1984. What would happen to sex crime over the following couple of decades as – in the language of the anti-porn movement – society was *bombarded* with a *torrent* of *extreme* material? What would the effects be on the USA, the leading nation in home-Internet adoption? What would happen as teenagers were able to access a diversity of online pornography with increasing ease?

What Happened Next?

The news media has always focused on the sensational, for at least one obvious reason: the public gets what the public wants, and the public has a great taste for scandal and disaster. The rising popularity of social media has, if anything, intensified the focus on the macabre and the titillating. As people have had increasing freedom in their choices of news sources, level-headed journalism has given way to click-bait - stories and headlines that are designed to grab the viewer's attention and generate ad revenue.

People do not, it appears, enjoy good news as much as bad; and yet the vast majority of the world's big stories in recent decades actually have fallen into this category. Stories of famine and deprivation hide the boring fact that global poverty has declined steeply in recent decades. Despite the steeply rising human population, the global proportion of people going hungry is almost certainly at its lowest level in history. The story of warfare is similar: the flood of tragic pictures from Syria, Libya or Sudan comes not because of a rise in global violence, but because the world is shrinking. These instant images brought to our smartphones and laptops mask the likely fact that fewer people today die violent deaths than ever before. According to the psychologist and writer Stephen Pinker in his recent book *The Better Angels of our Nature*, we run a lower risk of dying a violent death today than at any time in history.

It says something about human psychology, as well as the nature of political discussion, that few people are aware of these important facts, and that many reject them out-of-hand. We now have access to bad news from all over the world, so it often seems that bad news is everywhere. Besides our own gory fascination with such things, there are vested interests involved. Pictures of wounded or hungry children are useful for charity donations and interventionist governments; routine stories about the rapid decline of hunger in China, India or Nigeria are not.

When it comes to crime, it seems almost nobody is interested in good news: we love scare stories, and the media is more than happy to deliver them. Opposition politicians have an obvious incentive to exaggerate crime problems; furthermore, in an atmosphere where the public believes crime is rising, government ministers tend to be cautious in defending a record of falling crime, for fear of being attacked as not-tough-enough. Police forces, anxious to defend their budgets, will often play down successes and focus instead on crimes that are increasing. It is therefore unsurprising that people tend to (usually rightly) believe crime is falling in their own local area while also believing (usually wrongly) that crime is rising elsewhere. We accept a pessimistic outlook, despite the fact that it conflicts with our own personal experience.

In 2006, the *Washington Post* ran a story titled "Statistics Show Drop in U.S. Rape Cases"[84], revealing that the Justice Department's National Crime Victimization Survey (America's most comprehensive crime measure) had recorded a monumental 85% fall in rape cases in the 25 years from 1979 until 2004. The incidence of reported rape had plummeted from 2.8 cases per thousand to 0.4 per thousand in the space of a single generation. Here was a highly significant story: to put it another way, hundreds of thousands of rapes per year were no longer taking place.

But the public imagination is rarely captured by a negative fact. An absence of rape is an abstract idea. The media cannot publish the names and faces of rapists or their victims, and the numbers involved – millions of attacks that had simply not occurred during the 80s, 90s and early-2000s – are hard to visualise. Large numbers of non-victims are of little interest to a media and public accustomed to daily shock-and-awe journalism: this is not news. Despite its significance, the story received little attention. Stories of rape allow details to be pored over; they feed into a fierce public appetite for gossip, and allow the characters of the accused and accuser to be dissected in glorious detail. For stories to appeal to the public, they need to feature real people – ideally celebrities. The 2014 allegations of rape against Bill Cosby by dozens of women fed perfectly into the media circus, and so received saturation coverage. The missing millions of rape victims in America did not.

Some of the people approached for comment by the *Washington Post* cast doubt on the numbers, but there could be little doubt that the rate of sexual violence had fallen by a high degree. Attempts to explain the numbers by claiming that victims were reluctant to report rapes were misguided: in fact, the likelihood of a rape being reported had gone *up*, not down, in the decades since the 1960s sexual revolution began to reduce the stigma of reporting sex crimes. The *Washington Post* article pointed to figures showing that unreported rapes had fallen from 69% of the total to 61% between 1996 and 2006.

A few years later, the downward trend was confirmed. A 2013 US Justice Department study[85] recorded an even more astonishing decline in rape of 64% in a mere decade, from 1995 until 2005, after which the graph flattened out.

Why Has Rape Declined So Much?

The 2006 *Washington Post* report examined some possible reasons for the fall: perhaps a decline in hard-drug use, or tougher prison sentences. Alternatively, perhaps, better teaching of the issues around consent. However, the newspaper conspicuously failed to notice a key correlation: the post-1979 decline coincided with the arrival of home video recorders, and the steeper fall from 1995 onward exactly matched the arrival of home Internet connections.

Law professor Anthony D'Amato had long taken an interest in the issue, ever since being appointed in 1970 as a consultant to President Nixon's Commission on Obscenity and Pornography. D'Amato was unsurprised by the steep decline reported in 2006, and subsequently published a paper titled *Porn Up, Rape Down*, in which he expressed little doubt as to why reported rape had declined so steeply:

Official explanations for the unexpected decline include (1) less lawlessness associated with crack cocaine; (b) women have been taught to avoid unsafe situations; (c) more would-be rapists already in prison for other crimes; (d) sex education classes telling boys that "no means no." But these minor factors cannot begin to explain such a sharp decline in the incidence of rape.

There is, however, one social factor that correlates almost exactly with the rape statistics. The American public is probably not ready to believe it. My theory is that the sharp rise in access to pornography accounts for the decline in rape. The correlation is inverse: the more pornography, the less rape.

D'Amato looked beyond the national statistics to examine those at individual state level. The four states with the lowest Internet access were Arkansas, Kentucky, Minnesota and West Virginia. Far from matching the steep declines recorded across the country, these states actually bucked the trend and showed an *increase* in rape between 1980 and 2000.

He concluded:

Correlations aside, could access to pornography actually reduce the incidence of rape as a matter of causation? In my article I mentioned one possibility: that some people watching pornography may "get it out of their system" and thus have no further desire to go out and actually try it. Another possibility might be labeled the "Victorian effect": the more that people covered up their bodies with clothes in those days, the greater the mystery of what they looked like in the nude. The sight of a woman's ankle was considered shocking and erotic. But today, internet porn has thoroughly de-mystified sex. Times have changed so much that some high school teachers of sex education are beginning to show triple-X porn movies to their students in order to depict techniques of satisfactory intercourse.

Denying Good News

When it comes to the hugely emotive – and politicised – issue of rape, there is constant pressure to ignore good news. In the wake of the 1960s social revolutions, well-funded anti-rape organisations sprang up to campaign for legal and cultural changes around sexual violence. Logically, as a problem declines, one would expect resources to be redirected where they may be more urgently needed; but once vested interests have come into being, they will fight tooth-and-nail to maintain their funding and power. Additionally, as we have seen, sections of the feminist movement and the religious right vociferously argue that the 'pornification' of culture is driving an increase in sexual violence; a long-term decline is, therefore, inconvenient to their cause.

Thus, anti-rape organisations (or more accurately, bodies that *started out* as anti-rape organisations) are increasingly incentivised to deny the change in culture, to stretch the definition of sexual assault ever further by blurring the most serious with less serious crimes.

The Canadian columnist Margaret Wente refers to these vested interests as the 'grievance industry':

good news has been virtually ignored. Progressive people are right to deplore the supreme illogic of the [Canadian] government for cracking down on crime at a time when every type of major crime has hit historic lows. Yet other progressives insist that violence against women remains a serious problem...

The evidence is overwhelming. We are more enlightened now, and men – most men, anyway – behave much better. That is bad news for the grievance industry, which must stretch its definitions of assault and abuse to ridiculous extremes to keep its numbers up. It can't acknowledge the good news, because it has too much at stake.[86]

The Czech Story

So far, we have seen that in the most sexually liberal European countries, sexual violence declined following the legalisation of pornography; in America, the decline in rape correlates with the introduction of new technologies that made porn easier to access. Another interesting case study relates to the Czech Republic, which saw a sharp historical fracture in 1989, when the communist government fell, democracy was introduced, and many communist-era laws were repealed. At the start of the year, the Czech state had been among the world's most repressive; by December, it was one of the most liberal. Within a matter of months, the population saw state controls lifted and the introduction of free markets in – among other things – pornography. As with other states liberated from dictatorship, the new republic was extremely wary of any form of state intervention, and censorship controls were largely scrapped.

Here was a far more abrupt change than had been experienced in Denmark or the United States, and it affected many aspects of daily life. Pornography in communist Czechoslovakia was difficult and risky to obtain: now, suddenly, it was freely available, and completely uncensored. A 2010 paper titled *Pornography and Sex Crimes in the Czech Republic*[87] examined the resultant effects on sexual violence.

With the sudden removal of strict policing, overall crime rates quickly soared: the rate of non-sexual crime almost doubled overnight, and then plateaued for over a decade, before starting a rapid decline again. By 2009, it had fallen almost back to 1989 levels. However, sexual crime saw no such rise, remaining at about the same level as in communist times, and steadily drifting downwards thereafter. A more detailed look at sex crime by category revealed that, immediately following the revolution (and the introduction of porn), child sex abuse plummeted by almost half. It then quickly recovered to its original level, but has been in gradual long-term decline since. The study notes however that the nature of child sex crime changed after the revolution, which distorted the figures:

> The striking rise in reported child sex abuse depicted for the last half decade of the 1990s, according to notations and records in the Year Book of Ministry of Internal Affairs, do not apparently relate to the same types of child sex abuse recorded previously or afterward. They are believed to more closely reflect a concerted effort by the government to deal with a rise in child prostitution and the influx of foreign pimps, their prostitutes, and clients following the introduction of capitalism. This phenomenon seemed to be caused by the new economic situation and the society's attempt to cope. Once the child prostitution surge was dealt with, the downward trend in overall reports of child sex abuse continued.

The Czech Republic showed the same trend as elsewhere: no rise in sex crime associated with the rapid introduction of pornography, and signs of the exact opposite. In particular, the availability of porn correlates, in multiple studies, with a decline in the most serious sex crimes: child sex abuse and rape.

When Feminism and Science Collide

To understand why porn-viewing might be linked to a decline in sexual violence, it is worth visiting some simple questions about sex itself. Sex is such a deeply politicised subject that, despite the fact one can find 'expert' comment everywhere, few people understand the most basic aspects of our sexual behaviours. Sex has always been a subject where the science clashes with deeply-held feelings, and so the science of sex regularly comes under attack for reasons of superstition and dogma. The rapid recent decline of religion has (unfortunately) not been matched by a rise in scientific literacy. New, God-free myths about sex have been created to replace the old religious ones.

This was perfectly illustrated when I participated in a 2015 porn debate at Cambridge Union. Three comments from participants summed up the current mythology surrounding sex, even among those presenting themselves as experts. A student speaking from the floor demanded I apologise for claiming a correlation between porn-viewing and a decline in rape; then, an anti-porn speaker pointed out that the vast majority of rapes are committed by men, and presented this as evidence of insidious patriarchal influences; and finally, a pro-porn feminist speaker declared that the world could never be equal until women watched as much porn as men.

All three statements are based on the same popular myth: that differences in sexual behaviour between men and women are entirely social rather than biological in origin, and can therefore be 'fixed' – in much the same way that the American religious right declares homosexuality to be a choice, and therefore curable. Just as religious zealots cannot imagine a God who would create homosexuals, so certain feminists cannot tolerate a Mother Nature who would make men and women in any way different from each other.

The demand that I apologise for mentioning the reverse correlation between rape and porn was not issued on the basis that my information was inaccurate. My crime was far more serious than one of merely getting my facts wrong: I had blasphemed. It has become an article of feminist faith that 'rape is about violence, not sex'. The student's reasoning was correct: if (as she had been taught) rape is primarily motivated by a misogynistic desire to harm women, implanted in young men's minds by an entrenched system of patriarchal oppression, then porn-aided masturbation should not result in a steep decline in rape. Here was a classic problem: fact clashing with dogma, the unstoppable force meeting the immovable object.

There is, of course, no contradiction between human biology

and the classic feminist demand for equal rights. Whether or not men and women are biologically different is irrelevant: equal rights are an ethical construct, not a natural one, and do not depend on people being identical. However, once equal rights had been won in law by the mid-70s, sections of the left set out to go further and demand equal outcomes. This required a belief that significant biological differences between sexes did not exist, which set feminism – or at least some strands of feminism – on the course from political movement to religious one. Now, any scientific research finding differences must, of necessity, be denounced as heresy.

There were even (for a while in the 1970s) claims that physical differences in strength and agility between men and women were socially constructed, and that the coming fall of Patriarchy would result in women matching male sporting achievements. These ideas were in part aided by an astonishing rise in female athletic performance. But this, it transpired, was primarily down to heavy drug use among female athletes, especially those from Eastern European countries. Many female world records set in that era – such as the 800m record set in 1983 by a Czech runner – have never since been broken, and probably never will be.[88]

The theory of evolution by natural selection, developed by Charles Darwin and Alfred Russell Wallace in the 19th century, provided a huge challenge to established thinking. It is fun to mock creationists who deny evolution in its entirety, but more subtle – and fashionable – forms of evolution denial are alive and well today. While most educated people today accept that our bodies are the result of evolution, many are still unsettled by the idea that our minds also are, at least in part. The belief that human behaviour – including sex differences – might partly be driven by biology is sneeringly dismissed as 'biological determinism'.

For example, when I once tweeted an interesting but apparently uncontroversial science article comparing certain mating behaviours of bears to those of humans, a well-known sex blogger responded that "Biological determinism is a load of fucking bollocks!" – illustrating both the superstitious, ancient fear of the idea that humans are actually animals, as well as the nature of online debate on such subjects. It has become heresy to suggest that our behaviours are shaped by anything other than culture, despite the fact that the science in this area is well developed and is all but certain that genes do play a major role in human behaviour.

Since the human genome was decoded in 2003, it has become far easier to accurately separate the biological and environmental influences on our behaviours: the general conclusion is that almost all behaviours encapsulate both genetic and environmental components. To deny the role of evolution in sexual differences is to deny established science, but – worryingly – science-denial has once again become popular. Responding to this trend in 2010, the scientist and author Simon Baron-Cohen wrote:

> rejecting biological determinism makes no sense. We don't want to revert to the 1960s view that human behaviour is purely culturally determined, since we now know that view was profoundly mistaken. No one disputes that culture is important in explaining sex differences, but it can't be the whole story.[89]

Evolution denial has made a comeback, even as religion has gone into steep decline. This is one of a number of examples where 'liberal' thought and science have parted company in recent decades. In this and other ways, science denial is becoming mainstream on the left of politics, as it was once better associated with the religious right. The counter-Enlightenment, left or right, abhors Reason.

Equal rights have become confused with equal outcomes, as

illustrated by the strange suggestion at Cambridge Union that gender equality must require women and men to be equally inclined to watch pornography. But women and men will probably never be equally interested in pornography. The imbalance that causes this 'inequality' originates millions of years in our past, is embedded in our genes, and cannot be banished by political demands. To explain why, it is worth asking a question that is so fundamental we often forget to ask it.

What Is Sex?

To illustrate how little sex is understood, consider the question: What are the general, cross-species definitions of 'male' and 'female'? Such a simple question should be easy to answer, and yet few people can do so. In recent years, simply to ask the question has become akin to blasphemy. But how can we talk about pornography without understanding sex? To answer the question, we have to go back a billion years or so to the evolution of sexual intercourse.

Asexual reproduction – cloning – is simple: individuals create genetically identical copies of themselves, and the copies copy themselves, and so on. The problem with this is it creates no diversity. A disease that can kill one individual can sweep through a population of identical individuals and wipe it out. So sex evolved as a fix to the problem of uniformity.

Sexual reproduction involves combining genes from two individuals of the same species; this process is random, so that every new individual contains a unique combination of genes, and overall the population is diverse. Populations containing a lot of diversity are more likely to survive changes in the environment, from the appearance of a new disease or predator, to climate change. Sexual reproduction became widespread in nature because it makes species far more resilient.

Sexual species produce reproductive cells known as gametes (in humans, for example, these are eggs and sperm). Sexual reproduction involves the meeting of two gametes to form a new individual. The early sexes would have differed little from each other: to reproduce, a gamete of one sex would need to meet one of the other sex.

Gametes contain two useful things: genes (which describe how to build a new creature), and nutrition to give the 'baby' a start in life. Over time, one of the sexes – we can call it A – evolved a lazy strategy, and produced smaller gametes containing less nutrition. As a result, sex B was forced to produce ever bigger gametes to make up the difference. A became increasingly selfish, producing ever smaller gametes, which meant it could produce more of them. In response, B's gametes had to become ever larger, and fewer.

We call A male, and B female. Males make smaller gametes (sperm are the smallest cells in the human body), females make larger ones (eggs are our largest cells). A useful definition of female is therefore: it is the sex that invests most heavily in reproduction; and male is the sex that invests least. From this fairly small evolutionary change, hundreds of millions of years ago, emerge significant differences in male and female behaviours, across all sexual species.

In humans, these definitions obviously hold true. Women invest enormously in reproduction compared to men: they endure nine months of pregnancy, which requires extra food to be found, and puts women at additional health risk; then childbirth, which (prior to modern medicine) was often fatal; and then breastfeeding, which requires hundreds of extra calories per day. This huge cost to women clearly dwarfs the male investment: a few millilitres of semen.

On the surface then, females (of all species) lost the evolutionary war of the sexes, but in fact they had only lost the first battle. Males – with their lazy reproductive strategy – were now available to mate far more frequently than females. This imbalance allowed females, not males, to set the terms for mating. Female adaptations often included demanding payment in exchange for sex – in the form of food, security or nest-building for example. Males, freed from the cost of reproduction, were instead forced to devote their time and energy to courtship, or competing and fighting with other males, in order to prove themselves worthy mates. So another valid definition of the sexes is: female sex has high (relative) value, male sex has low value.

This imbalance expresses itself in different ways across species. In some of the most bizarre examples, many spiders and insects exhibit sexual cannibalism: males (and it is always males) offer their lives in exchange for the chance to mate. The opportunity for the male to fertilise a female is worth more than staying alive, and the female receives a good meal in exchange for offering sex: this is sexual commerce at its most brutal. Although this example is extreme, similar differences exist in many others species, and sexual commerce is widespread in nature – including, as we well know, in our own species.

Both sexual commerce and forced sex are common in the animal kingdom, and in almost all cases the roles are the same. Where sex is traded, it is females that sell and males that buy; and where forced sex happens, it is committed by males. Where humans differ from other animals, it is in the sophistication of our economic systems rather than our innate sexual behaviours. This was neatly demonstrated by accident during a research project into the economic behaviour of monkeys.

In 2005, Keith Chen, an economist at Yale, was conducting an experiment to determine whether capuchin monkeys could learn the concept of money, and if so, how sophisticated their financial behaviours might be. He painstakingly taught the monkeys how to exchange currency (a round metal disk with a hole in the middle) for different types of food with varying sugar content. Once they had learned the basics, he watched for various types of behaviour to evolve. He observed a range of interesting behaviours, and discovered that monkey speculators made similar mistaken assumptions to human investors (a fact that might not surprise many people who watch the stock market). However, perhaps his most interesting discovery was purely accidental: male monkeys learned to trade coins for sex with females. Chen had invented the monkey brothel (though one suspects that is not the way he would like to be remembered).

Too Many Men

Evolution has left human society with a problem, and bit by bit we are resolving it. Much of the world's great art and literature exists because of this problem, but it was perhaps most straightforwardly expressed by the UK grime artist Skepta:

> We need some more girls in here
> We need some more girls in here
> We need some more girls in here
> We need some more girls in here
> There's too many man too many many man
> Too many man too many many man
> Too many man too many many man
> Too many man too many many man

Unless we start genetically engineering our species, or decide to carry out selective abortion of male foetuses, there will always be too many men, from a reproductive standpoint at least. In humans, it is the female that selects mates, and a large part of human evolution is driven by sexual selection: which men (and so which genes) are selected by females for mating, and which are rejected. For men, the chance to reproduce is unfairly distributed: favoured males get to father disproportionate numbers of children with multiple partners, while many males lose out, and never reproduce at all. In crude economic terms, there is a vast overproduction of sperm in the world – or alternatively a huge shortage of eggs – and this is the root cause of many problems.

Society has developed various solutions to lessen the imbalance and so promote stability: social monogamy made life fairer (under the system of polygyny, more typical in ancient times, females would choose to mate with the most socially powerful males, even if they already had mates); prostitution – certainly the oldest profession – provides an outlet for men without mates. And pornography makes masturbation more exciting and satisfying, which provides a harmless way to deal with unneeded sperm. As Anthony D'Amato wrote in *Porn Up, Rape Down*: "some people watching pornography may 'get it out of their system' and thus have no further desire to go out and actually try it".

What Might Happen if Porn is Banned?

The powerful evidence that easy porn access is linked with reduced sexual violence can be applied in reverse. What might happen if the unprecedented open access to the Internet, taken for granted for decades, becomes restricted – as now seems to be happening?

The American sexual psychologist and author Dr David J Ley believes Britain's censorious path will inevitably lead us into trouble.

Does interfering with masturbation and private sexual stimulation have larger social effects? Apparently, we shall now see... I'm sad to say that the people of the United Kingdom may need to get out your rape whistles, and attend personal defense classes.[90]

A 2006 paper titled *Pornography, Rape and the Internet* by Todd D Kendal[91] agreed that porn appeared to reduce rape, especially among teenagers. Kendall found that in America, "states that adopted the internet quickly saw larger declines in rape incidence than other states (while no similar effect is evident for homicide)" and an especially profound effect on young men: "I find a significant negative effect of internet access on rape arrest rates among men ages 15-19 – a group for whom pornography was most restricted before the internet".

In a nutshell, preventing teenagers from accessing pornography – as British politicians and regulators are determined to do – seems highly likely to cause a spike in sexual violence, and reverse much of the progress made against rape in recent years. It is time to turn the tables on the porn panic. It is the anti-sex movement, with its false arguments for censorship, that poses the greatest risks, especially to young women.

9

Free Expression on the Edge

Don't you see that the whole aim of Newspeak is to narrow the range of thought? In the end we shall make thoughtcrime literally impossible, because there will be no words in which to express it – George Orwell, *1984*

My journey from left-wing activist to technologist to porn vendor to free-speech campaigner has been an endlessly fascinating one. I have always been of a broadly liberal mindset (with a small L), with a natural distrust of authoritarians, though would never have referred to myself as a liberal during my Marxist days. The far-left's leanings towards authoritarianism always tended to leave me somewhat cold, and help to explain why I drifted away from tribal activism, while still retaining many of those ideals.

But free speech did not feature often in left-wing campaigning, and I was never close to the anti-censorship movement, if there ever really was such a thing in Britain. In practise, the great battles for free expression – such as *Lady Chatterley's Lover* – have been left to individual artists, writers and publishers choosing to bravely stick their heads above the parapet and challenge the wisdom of the status quo; or (very occasionally) to politicians like Roy Jenkins, for whom liberty was more than a vague, nice-to-have concept. Like many people, I assumed there were good people out there, fighting the good fight for all of us.

It was in 2011 when I awoke to the real, pressing threat to something we have all come to take for granted: free access to the Internet, a medium that has wrought fundamental, lasting change to human culture. As Chair of the Adult Industry Trade

Association (AITA), I was invited to be a witness at a parliamentary enquiry, called by the Tory MP Claire Perry, on 'online safety for children' – something that had now become an established euphemism for censorship. The process left me feeling despondent: it consisted of four short sessions held over two days. I gave evidence at one, and sat in on another, and witnessed a huge abuse of due process, as well as of reason.

Witness after witness provided their view that porn was leading children to sexually assault each other in the playground, or that teens were committing gang rape as the result of watching it. None of the testimony I saw was backed by research or any specific detail. Some of it was entertaining: for example, the ex-Labour Home Secretary Jacqui Smith's insistence that porn was leading people to try anal sex. She failed to clarify why this was a bad thing, or note that anal sex has been popular at least since God destroyed Sodom and Gomorrah; but the MPs sitting on the committee showed a lack of curiosity.

Predictably, Perry's enquiry came up with the recommendation that ISPs should provide child-safe filters, and force all home-Internet subscribers to make a decision to opt in or out of the system. These were brought into being in early 2014, not because of a new law, but as a result of David Cameron arm-twisting the major ISPs into voluntarily implementing the system. The rollout was a farce, as the filters were found to cover far more than pornography – both by design and by accident. When ISPs refused to allow public access to the list of blocked sites, the Open Rights Group built its own software to probe networks and determine which sites had been blocked, and discovered that Sky, one of the largest UK ISPs, was blocking 19 percent of all websites in its filter.[92]

No wonder less than ten percent of subscribers had enabled the filters anyway[93]: this fact was used by future anti-porn campaigns to prove just how irresponsible British parents were, and that therefore the state should act to protect children both from the evils of pornography and their own permissive parents.

The enquiry showed me that almost nobody was defending expression on principle – least of all, 'indefensible' expression such as pornography. After I gave evidence, a Tory MP approached me and shook my hand, saying he had never heard anybody defend porn before, nor even believed that was possible.

As my campaigning developed, I increasingly came to see porn censorship as just a special case of a more general problem. It was undoubtedly true that sexual expression was feared in its own right, but this fear was being used by the authorities to justify censorship that had really very little to do with either porn or child protection. There is little point in opposing censorship in one case while ignoring it in another, as the end result is the same: an unaccountable and non-transparent bureaucracy with the power to block content as it chooses.

Not long ago, such a system was the realm of governments in China, Iran or Saudi Arabia. Now its implementation is possibly imminent in the UK, and the press, having been told it is merely a mechanism to protect children from pornography, has showed a near-total lack of curiosity. One rare journalist who had been trying unsuccessfully to pitch the ATVOD story to the press confided in me: "Discouragingly hard to get people onside once the word porn comes into it. I'm surprised and irritated by it."

End of the Porn Panic?

For authoritarians within the state, porn was merely one of the excuses to construct a system of Internet censorship, and the anti-sex protagonists of the porn panic had provided them cover. By late-2015, the earlier anti-sex feminist groups had faded. UK Feminista appeared to have become dormant, while Object simply closed its website one day.

Why did they fizzle out? Partly because they had lost the arguments. The hard evidence against sexual expression had never been produced, and the public continued to remain remarkably unpanicked. In part, they faded because a less extreme-sounding body had taken over the campaign. Child's Eye Line UK continued the work of the earlier groups using more sober, less extreme language, and focusing exclusively on the 'threat to children'. They did not provide any more evidence of harm than any of the other groups, but they did not need to. To say "Sure, we have nothing against nude imagery, but do we really want children to see it?" was a more effective argument than trying to claim the porn industry is invading our brains or creating an imaginary rape epidemic.

Child's Eye Line's named supporters were drawn from across the political spectrum, from religious groups, unions and charities. The supportive MPs listed on their website came from all parties, but were skewed leftward, heavy in Labour MPs, as well as from the Green Party and Scottish National Party, while once such a campaign would have been heavy in Tories. Buried among the list of individual supporters were some usual suspects: anti-sex feminists such as Gail Dines and the comedian Kate Smurthwaite. The Think-Of-The-Children message masked a simple truth: it is impossible to 'protect children' from any exposure to nude or erotic imagery without also 'protecting' adults from it.

The porn panic also faded because, in large part, its job was done. The drive to censor the Internet had now moved within Parliament and within government. Multiple attempts to introduce a blocking law had already failed, but the next attempt would probably gain government backing. By late-2015, the Online Safety Bill was making its way through the House of Lords: this was a tough censorship bill sold as a simple child-protection one. And whether or not this bill failed, it was widely expected that an Internet censorship bill would be announced in the Queen's Speech in the Spring.

But most of all, the arguments had simply moved on from sex.

Rising fear of terrorism and political extremism had transformed the political landscape. Only a few years before, discussion of political censorship would have been unacceptable, so porn provided a useful proxy. Now, political censorship was on the agenda, and was becoming accepted across the political spectrum.

The arguments for censorship had been honed to suit each target audience. For some, terrorist attacks provide an excellent excuse for blocking 'terrorist content': in the authoritarian hands of Home Secretary Theresa May, this had broadened into a commitment to censor 'extremist content', which is an ominously unspecific term. For the authoritarian right, censorship of 'Muslim extremists' was now acceptable.

For those who liked to see themselves as more liberal, other excuses worked better: the already vague concept of 'hate speech' had become broadened to encapsulate any speech that might cause offence; and this could mean almost any speech at all. Depressingly, the case for censorship had been made, and opposition was close to non-existent on both right and left. In Parliament, the liberal conscience had previously been repre-sented by a small group of Liberal Democrat MPs; but these had been almost wiped out in the May 2015 election. Beyond them, free expression was seen as nothing more than a hobby for eccentrics such as the Tory MP David Davis.

Outside Parliament, a new generation was determined to shut down speech on an unprecedented scale. The erosion of liberal values in universities was one of the most worrying signs of the change to British political culture, and a warning that the new culture of authoritarianism would become even deeper in coming years.

No Platform

In the 1970s, student unions began a policy of No Platform For Fascism, specifically excluding violent, anti-democratic far-right groups a platform for promoting their views on university campuses. As an anti-fascist campaigner in the 80s, I supported this narrowly drawn form of censorship, though, like many anti-fascists, I have since changed my mind for several reasons.

For many of us, the tipping point came in 2009 when Nick Griffin, leader of the British National Party was invited to appear on BBC TV's *Question Time*. It was unprecedented for a far-right figure to be given such a powerful platform. I was among several thousand people outside the studios protesting against the BBC's decision. But Griffin's appearance did not lead to a spike in support for the BNP, nor an increase in racial violence. In fact, it exposed Griffin for what he was: a mere human being, with simplistic, outdated ideas that were easy to challenge and dismantle. Far from aiding the British far-right, the programme helped create the conditions for the BNP's decline and Griffin's downfall.

Here was a lesson in an old Enlightenment concept: John Stuart Mills' marketplace of ideas, in which all speech should be allowed, but open debate would, in time, sift the good ideas from the bad, the right from the wrong. Possibly Griffin had been aided rather than harmed by his former pariah status: in being labelled as too dangerous for public consumption, his racist, nationalistic and anti-immigrant beliefs had been elevated to a level of importance that they did not deserve.

No Platform For Fascism had additional problems. Once a far-right party like the BNP begins to play by the rules of democracy and win council seats, then to deny it a platform is an anti-democratic act. At a stroke, an anti-fascist policy becomes a quasi-fascist one. Political censorship is exposed for what it is: an act of fascism, not something that should be embraced by progressives.

Unfortunately, the student left did not appear to have read Mills. Rather than abandon No Platform For Fascism, it expanded a thousand-fold to become simply No Platform, and in the new era of intolerance, was wielded against a bewildering array of targets. No Platform generally means a refusal to host a speaker, though it can be implemented by simply shouting down 'unacceptable' individuals or ideas. It is deeply unintelligent, even childish behaviour, and it has become widespread in academia.

Targets of No Platform have included the radical feminist Julie Bindel, who had long ago written a *Guardian* article considered to be transphobic, and so was barred from multiple student unions, even when discussing issues that had nothing to do with transsexual politics. I witnessed this first-hand when I debated pornography with her at the University of Essex, and a petition was circulated trying to ban her. I was amused that the students were attacking the anti-porn feminist rather than me, the evil defender of patriarchal oppression. The petition failed, but Bindel was met with a fierce protest outside the debate, and was clearly shaken by it.

A sign that politics has become dangerously toxic is that it places itself beyond parody. In October 2015, Manchester University Students' Union banned both speakers from a planned debate on censorship.[94] Julie Bindel was (again) excluded for her allegedly 'transphobic' views. Her opponent, the right-wing gay libertarian journalist Milo Yiannapoulos was then banned for being an alleged 'misogynist', as well as other thoughtcrimes. It had become impossible to discuss censorship on campus, because those who opposed censorship were being labelled extremists.

Does It Matter?

In 2010, I became worried about an apparent increase in far-right activity, and decided to return to activism, this time as a blogger and social-media user. I created the persona MoronWatch, and took aim at the BNP's Nick Griffin, and others on the British and American right, as well as creationists, gun advocates, astrologers, homeopathy practitioners and other assorted people that I felt were worth mocking. I still strongly identified as left-wing.

In hindsight, but not by design, MoronWatch was a unique character. Instead of blocking 'dangerous' people, I followed them. Instead of screaming 'racist!', 'homophobe!' and other terms of abuse, I mocked them gently, encouraged others to join the fun, and created a popular Twitter persona that quickly attracted thousands of left-wing and liberal followers.

When the anti-Islamic, far-right English Defence League was born, I dedicated a good deal of MoronWatch effort to mocking and exposing them. I felt that here was something that had not been seen in many years: a far-right street movement that could attract thousands to a protest. I feared a fascist resurgence was underway, and set out to help tackle it. My approach was unusual: the standard anti-EDL clicktivist would seek out EDL supporters on Twitter, tell them they were racist scum, then block them. Instead, I would mock, tease but also – where possible – engage EDL supporters in discussion.

This was, after all, how the National Front was ultimately undermined in the early-1980s: through dialogue. White working-class people shared workplaces with non-whites, supported the same football teams and listened to the same reggae and ska music. Like black and Asian youth, young white working-class men faced police violence, especially outside football stadiums. The old left – via trade unions, Labour Party branches and football supporters' clubs, could bring communities together, and they were immensely successful in tackling the scourge of racism during the 1980s.

Engaging with EDL supporters taught me the same lesson. Many early supporters quickly walked away from the group in disgust, once its underlying racism and lies began to be exposed. Many had joined because they had seen large numbers of Pakistani and Bengali immigrants move into their neighbourhoods, and they felt threatened by the pace of change. In this, they were little different from more middle-class activists who later protested against 'gentrification' in trendy areas of London, but were not received with the same sympathy.

Other EDL supporters apparently joined simply for a social life. Coaches were chartered from working-class towns and estates to take supporters to each protest. Thanks to the wonder of Twitter, one could see them on their way to demonstrations, boasting about how many cans of beer they were bringing, how many lines of mephedrone or cocaine they had consumed on the way. Here were young, white, working-class people finding a rare opportunity to assemble and feel pride in their own beleaguered identities: hatred of the white working-class is, after all, the last acceptable prejudice.

And online, I began to feel uneasy about my own Twitter followers. I saw middle-class student leftists mocking working-class people for their poor spelling rather than their racist views, telling them they were scum; those EDL supporters who tried to explain why they were uneasy about immigration were told they were racists, and blocked. Many of those I spoke to were clearly not racists, though they had absorbed lies about Muslims that needed to be countered. How were we to defuse the EDL if we refused to speak to them?

In 2012, the EDL announced plans to march in Walthamstow, an area of east London with a large Muslim population, a few miles from the site of Oswald Mosley's 1936 defeat. Here was an opportunity to demonstrate community solidarity in the face of a fascist threat. Instead, the government – to cheers from anti-fascists – banned the march. But not just the EDL was affected: all marches were banned, for a month, in four London boroughs, including a planned anti-racist march.

So, the EDL had been elevated from an annoyance to a national threat, which no doubt helped its recruitment that month. The state's denial of its free speech fed into far-right conspiracy theories about a takeover of the state by 'cultural Marxism'. And the opportunity for anti-fascists to unite and offer a joyous display of cross-racial support for British Muslims was denied. All this might be fine, so long as we trust the state to always act progressively; and anybody who does is oblivious to the lessons of history.

After a rapid rise in support, EDL strength plateaued and then declined. It became clear that they were less the foundation of a mass movement and more an expression of working-class disenfranchisement. There was no longer any place in left-wing politics for white, working-class people, and so groups like the EDL provided an outlet for their frustrations.

Around that time, I awoke to the nature of the new left. I had encountered conservative feminism via my sex-industry work, and found to my discomfort that the pro-censorship left was now embedded in trade unions, the Labour and Green parties, local authorities and academia. The ideas I had supported all my life: women's rights, gay rights and opposition to racism – had now been seized on by mostly white, middle-class bullies as excuses to pillory people and attack free speech.

When gay marriage was voted on in Parliament, the minority that raised opposition online – typically older, more religious people – were told they were homophobes and fascists, and were silenced by the online mob. This bullying was ugly and unnecessary: there was a clear majority, in the country and in Parliament, in favour of gay marriage. An earlier generation would have been magnanimous in this victory, ignored the voices of the past and celebrated. Instead, the stench of witch-hunt was growing stronger, and again it was coming from the left.

Fascist methods were no longer confined to the political right, but had spread across the political spectrum. And while the far-right was as ugly as ever, it was gaining no significant base; but the authoritarian left had gained positions of true power: in the Labour Party, unions, the civil service, media regulators and academia. It had backing in the quality press. I came to the conclusion that the rise of fascism in Britain was going largely unchecked, because few recognised it as fascism.

Is It Fascism?

Fascism is often incorrectly applied to military dictatorships. Regimes such as Franco's in Spain, Pinochet's in Chile and Zia's in Pakistan have been mislabelled as fascist. Fascism is far more disturbing than military coups and state-initiated authoritarianism. It comes from below, not above; from the masses, not the government. It is a backlash by the most conservative tendencies in society. It can appear shrouded in religion, or as a secular force. It is always anti-intellectual, anti-science and anti-progress, though it can happily co-opt the language of science and progress.

Whether the left-wing counter-Enlightenment is fascist or not is partly a matter of semantics. The f-word is so overused that it is not particularly useful to deploy anyway. But the counter-Enlightenment movements of both left and right have become increasingly similar, and in many instances have begun to blur into one. Enlightenment values of Liberty, Equality, Reason are all under attack from assorted movements of both left and right.

Take migration for example. On the surface, anti-foreigner sentiment is focused on the right, while the left is nominally less prone to xenophobia. But in fact, the two strands have become intertwined. Left-wingers, for example, often now rail against the evil of *foreign* corporations and *foreign* bankers. The Marxist internationalism of my youth would not distinguish between foreign or local corporations; now the left-wing anti-corporate message has morphed subtly into a xenophobic one. The dubious movement against 'gentrification' in London has made it acceptable to rail against property purchase by *foreign* investors. As Colin Wiles pointed out in the *Guardian*, this narrative was inaccurate, and often masked anti-immigration sentiment: "Is a

French banker who has rented in London for 10 years and now decided to buy a foreigner or a Londoner?"[95] And as Dave Hill wrote, also in the *Guardian*, foreign buyers were less significant in property price rises than many were claiming:

> about 10,000 more people moved in to London from elsewhere (370,000) than moved out (360,000) – not much of a difference. So how come the capital's population is rising so incredibly fast, and has recently topped 8.3 million? Yes, it's the birth rate, stupid: 134,037 babies were born here in the year to mid-June 2012, according to the ONS estimate. This is a city that breeds.[96]

Left-wing commentators have also recently embraced the anti-sex-trafficking narrative, which in fact is a thinly veiled alliance between the old anti-prostitution and anti-immigration movements. This movement claims – falsely – that millions of women and girls (yes, always women and girls) are being dragged around the globe by the Patriarchy to be raped for profit. The myth provides police forces a cover to raid brothels, identify women working illegally (or 'trafficked women', as they are now called) and rescue them (i.e. hand them to immigration officers for detention and deportation). All of this is applauded by some feminists, and others on the left, including veteran campaigners, journalists and trade-unionists. As with the porn panic, a thin veneer of feminist rhetoric covers attitudes and actions more usually associated with the extreme right. (Readers with an interest in this area are advised to read Laura Agustín's 2007 book, *Migration, Labour Markets and the Rescue Industry*).

The anti-banker feeling that surfaced after the 2008 crash has happily merged with anti-Semitic sentiment, and when a blogger rails against Zionist bankers, it can be hard to place them on the political spectrum. Nouveau-leftist Russell Brand fell into this trap in October 2014 when he invited anti-bank activist Lawrence

Easeman to help launch his book, *Revolution*, only to learn that Easeman's online activism appeared to be tinged with anti-Semitic and pro-Nazi outbursts. Brand's book launch had to be postponed.

And as the left was appropriating right-wing ideas, so the far-right was doing the reverse. The EDL, and similar far-right groups in Europe, abandoned overt racism, homophobia and anti-Semitism, and appropriated progressive language to attack Muslims. Women's rights, gay rights, sexual freedom, secularism, female genital mutilation, 'honour killings' and belief in democracy were used to falsely paint Muslim immigrants as a threat to European values, including the Enlightenment. And many on the left, deliberately or inadvertently, joined the Muslim-bashing. Cruel, bullying attacks on Muslims, such as the 2010 French ban on veils, were often held up as successes for secularism or women's rights, while in fact they continued an old French tradition of intolerance for minorities. "The creatures outside looked from pig to man, and from man to pig, and from pig to man again; but already it was impossible to say which was which."

But You Can't Say That!

The critical point at the heart of defence of free speech is this: speech and physical behaviour are different things. Speech, and other expression, allows us to discuss, even joke about the most horrific things – murder, rape, torture, genocide – without any real people being killed, raped or tortured. There are very limited cases where speech could be said to be definitively harmful: a general ordering his troops to commit a massacre is clearly using speech to initiate something horrific, and can be held accountable in a war-crimes trial. But here, there are more issues more than mere words involved: soldiers are trained and paid to follow orders. They have pre-committed to obey whatever their leader commands them to do, and can be severely punished for not doing so. The words are not just words, they are orders.

Those who seek to ban speech must set out to show that it can be harmful in far broader cases; and since humans are not mere automatons who can be turned into violent zombies at the flick of a switch, this is not an easy task. Regardless of the claims made during moral panics, we do not watch porn and therefore commit rape, any more than we watch violent films and commit murder, or watch war movies and then go to war.

As seen earlier, the anti-sex movement set out to redefine harm by using porn-panic words – objectification and so on – to falsely paint sexual expression as dangerous to women and children. The same trick is now deployed by authoritarians to attack any form of expression, and again, it is primarily the political left that today defines the rules of censorship.

A new language has been developed to justify censorship on nominally liberal grounds, designed to blur the clear lines between speech and physical harm. Strange new words and concepts are invented to obfuscate discussions about expression.

Safe Spaces, Triggers and Cyber-Violence

Much of the new language for censorship appeared suddenly and recently, though much of it had been brewing in obscure corners of academia for some time.

I encountered 'safe spaces' in 2013, when the east London stripper activists – some of whom we met earlier in this book – launched their own body, the East London Stripper Collective, to promote and defend their art-form. On the Facebook event page for their launch party, one attendee asked whether it would be OK to bring a male friend, or whether this would violate a safe space?

We had suddenly re-entered an era in which it was acceptable to exclude people simply based on their sex, race or other attribute of birth. We had fast-rewound to the 1950s. The question was objectionable because it implied that all men were to be treated as potentially dangerous, even in the context of such a party. It was anyway ludicrous, because strippers take their clothes off safely in front of mostly male audiences on a daily basis.

The 'safe space' idea was appearing everywhere, and closely linked to pro-censorship feminism and identity politics. The more 'oppressed' a person might decide they were, the greater privilege they would be granted to exclude 'privileged' people from some event or place. The Geek Feminism Wiki defines it as follows:

> Safe space is a term for an area or forum where either a marginalised group are not supposed to face standard mainstream stereotypes and marginalisation, or in which a shared political or social viewpoint is required to participate in the space.[97]

The Victorian Lady, a nervous creature prone to bouts of hysteria in response to pretty much anything, was back. But instead of hysteria (a derivative of the Greek word for uterus), a new pseudo-scientific term was introduced: she could be *triggered*. The Geek Feminism Wiki explains:

> Trigger warnings are customary in some feminist and other Safe spaces. They are designed to prevent unaware encountering of certain materials or subjects for the benefit of people who have an extremely strong and damaging emotional response (for example, post-traumatic flashbacks or urges to harm themselves) to such topics. Having these responses is called "being triggered".[98]

Free-speech advocate and Canadian lesbian Katherine Cooper (I merely mention her 'oppressions' to bolster my argument to fans of identity politics) points out the dishonesty of the 'trigger warning' concept. It only applies to certain, pre-selected types of trigger. So in practise, it becomes a tool to reinforce existing prejudices, especially regarding sex. Recovering from PTSD, Cooper experiences trauma from:

> A specific Elvis Presley song, the number 54, and the scent of cafeteria kitchens. These things always cause me to feel panicky or short of breath. It would be ridiculous to expect some random stranger to know this. I can definitely understand general graphic content or discretion warnings but ANYTHING can be a trigger nowadays.

While, of course, anybody is at liberty to lock themselves in a soundproof room without an Internet connection to avoid any form of expression that might offend (or rather, trigger) them, the concept would inevitably broaden into the public sphere, and become a tool to justify the censorship of anything, anywhere. It was used, for example, as part of the justification to ban Page 3 of the *Sun* since now, train carriages and buses must become safe spaces, protected from pictures of breasts that may trigger anybody with nipple-anxiety.

Now that public spaces had been declared a threat to womenfolk, the idea of a return to women-only train carriages was even raised, and briefly caused a furore when Jeremy Corbyn was put on the spot, and refused to rule them out during his Labour leadership campaign. The carriages had been scrapped in 1977 following the introduction of equality legislation which had been a victory for the feminist movement. Equality, a cornerstone of the Enlightenment, and of 1960s liberalism, is now under ferocious attack from the left.

Once triggering and safe spaces became popular, at least in the fringes of feminism and the student left, these would inevitably extend themselves to online 'spaces'. And now, here was a language to justify the permanent, ongoing censorship of all dialogue. Discussion of anything deemed to be potentially 'triggering' must now be policed, whether by the self-appointed inquisition, or the state.

If triggering were not already justification enough to introduce unprecedented levels of speech policing, speech itself has been relabelled to make it seem scarier. 'Cyber-violence' is born. Now, one need not argue that words might, through some convoluted process, lead to violence: henceforth, words *are* violence.

This Orwellian use of language to attack the most basic forms of free speech is no longer the preserve of pro-censorship activists on university campuses. In September 2015, the United Nations Broadband Commission published a report advising governments to take urgent action to "combat online violence against women and girls".[99] The idea that words are violence is not explained nor questioned, simply stated.

The report launch event was attended by Anita Sarkeesian, a leading pro-censorship feminist voice, who explained that cyber-violence was not limited to death threats, but might include "the day-to-day grind of 'you're a liar' and 'you suck'". In other words, cyber-violence is nothing at all like violence, but is actually about people saying mean things to each other on the Internet.

Undeterred, the report's findings are designed to provoke moral panic: "almost three quarters of women online have been exposed to some form of cyber violence". A near-transparent call for draconian language-policing is made: governments are urged to "work harder and more effectively together to better protect the growing number of women and girls who are victims of online threats and harassment".

The fact that the report was specifically related to women and girls might imply that women were more likely than men to experience online violence: but in fact, as with violence of the real, non-cyber variety, the reverse is true. A Demos study of over two-million tweets sent to celebrities found that men received far more abuse than women online: one in 20 tweets to men were abusive compared to one in 70 for women.[100] Despite the popular 'massive online misogyny' narrative, the real problem is not that women are the target of more abuse than men, but that today's women are not considered capable (by pro-censorship feminists, at any rate) of dealing with it as men can. Equality would be nice, they seem to be saying, if only women weren't so easily triggered.

Where Do We Draw the Line?

Any discussion on liberty tends to focus on defining acceptable limits. John Stuart Mills provided a lasting, liberal response which he called the Harm Principle: that people's actions should only be constrained where they harm others.

Discussions of liberty and harm can be complex, but in the area of expression, they become relatively simple. Expression is never truly violent (unless you call it cyber-violence, that is). In almost three decades of online political discussion, I have been subject to pretty much every form of verbal and written insult known to man. I have also been physically assaulted (for unrelated reasons): only somebody who has no experience of violence would try to compare it to speech. Beyond direct incitement to violence, it is generally hard to make claims of harm stick.

Hate speech has become today's frontline for censorship, because hatred is widely hated. However, it is unlikely that most bans on hateful language can reduce hate, and very likely that censorship of hate speech can make things worse. Limiting hate speech necessarily limits the discussion of hate speech, since censors and police tend not to be subtle in distinguishing between the two. Once a discussion of a problem is taboo, solutions cannot be found. Online censorship is often automated, and thus even worse than the old-fashioned varieties. Mention of specific words or phrases can trigger acts of censorship without any regard to context; and the more censorious the climate, the less context matters anyway. Censors under orders to stop hate will act conservatively and remove more than necessary.

Censorship of hate speech tends to ignore how humans actually behave. The throwing of insults may be unpleasant, but in fact is often a first step *away* from violence, rather than a step towards it. This is a benefit of expression – it allows us to rehearse terrible things without causing actual harm. Exchanges of insulting words may just as easily lead to more pleasant interchanges as to violence. Words provide a safe way for people – who may indeed hate each other – to interact.

Insulting words may not actually be insulting at all. As a Jew, I personally have no problem with Spurs fans calling themselves 'Yiddos'. This football chant is not directed at Jews, nor meant as an insult, but because the word, in other contexts, is insulting, it is labelled a hate term. In late-2013, police warned Spurs fans they could face arrest for chanting it. Furthermore, discussion of the police threat was censored in the media, leading to headlines such as: "Tottenham in talks with police over 'Y' word arrest threat" in the *Evening Standard*.

While it is impossible to see how these police threats could reduce anti-Semitic hatred in any way, they could certainly aid the far-right by feeding into their idea that Jews are subject to special treatment, and most dangerously they suppress the discussion of important and sensitive issues. This is a tragedy, because one of the greatest tools in tackling bigotry is humour; and now, 'offensive' comedy is increasingly subjected to censorship. As a Jew, I would much rather know who hates me or my family, and be given the opportunity to respond and educate people with bigoted views. I have, more than once, corrected anti-Semitic myths that friends have believed and repeated. To silence such people denies me the opportunity to challenge their ideas. Censorship designed to protect me actually disempowers me.

I have increasingly grown to admire the way in which America tolerates hateful speech that would be censored in much of Europe, and there are valuable lessons to be learned from the US. By leaving difficult but non-violent situations to communities to resolve, rather than to police, unexpected and often happy outcomes can occur.

The Westboro Baptist Church provides a prime example of this. The church is a vile little family business based in Kansas, which excels in trolling to create outrage, and thus publicity for itself. The address of WBC's website tells much of the story: godhatesfags.com. WBC goes out of its way to troll targets that are guaranteed to provoke shock, and is famous for protesting at the funerals of dead soldiers returning from Iraq and Afghanistan, as well as the funerals of the victims of mass shootings. Its thesis is that all of these deaths are God's punishment against America for tolerating homosexuality.

It is tempting to wish that the police would simply intervene and stop them upsetting bereaved families, but so long as they stay on public land, they are protected by the First Amendment. An equivalent organisation in Britain would quickly face arrest and imprisonment on a variety of pretexts, and I would once have applauded that.

But a key reason for the protection of free speech is that it empowers citizens to provide innovative solutions that are more intelligent, harmonious, humorous and long-lasting than the simplistic and unimaginative use of state power.

Mills' free marketplace of ideas would suggest that the community should be left to find its own responses. In the absence of state intervention against WBC, how could the people themselves resolve the situation, without resorting to violence or other illegal behaviour? Since 2005, a voluntary group of bikers called the Patriot Guard Riders has attended funerals to prevent them being disrupted by WBC. The riders form a shield between mourners and protesters, and when necessary drown out the shouts of WBC pickets by singing, or revving their bike engines. They also attend the funerals of homeless veterans who might otherwise not be mourned. The state's protection of WBC's free speech created the space for an inspiring show of human kindness. Human problems require human responses, not the smothering security blanket preferred by the British state.

I do not claim that the PGR is in any way perfect, or that its response is the best one: as an internationalist I wince at the word 'patriot', for example. Most likely, like all human organisations, it will degrade into something other than it was intended for. But provided free-speech protections remain, the community will find solutions to that new problem, if it ever happens.

Back in Britain, the EDL was eclipsed by a far bigger threat from the right. UKIP, though not a purely far-right organisation, certainly attracted support from the disparate far-right as well as disenfranchised working-class ex-Labour and Conservative voters. The party demonstrated the worthless nature of 'hate speech' protections, and circumnavigated the rules with ease. UKIP's leader Nigel Farage became adept at 'dog whistle' politics: making statements that breached none of the rules of British state censorship, while still attacking minority groups.

Because speech censorship is necessarily a dumb, brute-force endeavor, it is easy to break. There is nothing to be gained in today's British politics by overtly attacking a racial group, as might have happened regularly until the 1980s. Instead, Farage chose to suggest that immigrants with HIV were causing problems for the National Health Service. The implication is clear: foreigners are bringing disease. If he had said that overtly, he may have breached hate-speech laws. But the statement was partly truthful, so difficult to ban as 'hate'. Statistically, immigrants *are* more likely to have HIV than British-born people. However, the idea that the NHS was struggling to cope was nonsense – the problem is miniscule compared to the NHS budget, and it would probably cost more to exclude people with HIV than treat them (as well as being deeply immoral). But Farage's point did its job for him far more effectively than if he had used crude – and criminalised – racial slurs.

Censorship of hate speech does nothing to curb any future fascist threat, but it does prevent open discussion of community problems and community solutions to them. Ultimately the idea of 'good censorship' is a fallacy. It is physically and logically impossible to construct a system that keeps out all the 'bad stuff' while allowing the 'good stuff' to get through. In fact, simply finding a universally agreed definition of 'good' and 'bad' would be impossible.

The US Supreme Court judge Louis Brandeis wrote in 1927 that censorship regimes cannot stay ahead of threats to liberty:

> Those who won our independence by revolution were not cowards. They did not fear political change. They did not exalt order at the cost of liberty. To courageous, self-reliant men, with confidence in the power of free and fearless reasoning applied through the processes of popular government, no danger flowing from speech can be deemed clear and present, unless the incidence of the evil apprehended is so imminent that it may befall before there is opportunity for full discussion. If there be time to expose through discussion the falsehood and fallacies, to avert the evil by the processes of education, the remedy to be applied is more speech, not enforced silence.

Or as it is often summarised: the solution to bad speech is more speech.

From 1984 to 2016

The United Kingdom is on course to become the first democratic country to introduce a large-scale regime of website-blocking.

While there is an endless parade of justifications for this – from preventing terrorism to protecting women from being insulted on Twitter – the vehicle for delivering this censorship will most likely be the protection of children from pornography. Yet porn is not harmful: its availability appears to have, on balance, a beneficial effect on society.

Meanwhile, British liberalism is at its lowest ebb in decades. There are few voices in the public sphere prepared to declare censorship a very un-British thing to do. The Human Rights Act, which contains a protection of free expression in Article 10 (if a fairly weak one) is under threat from the Conservatives; and even if it survives, the UK's membership of the EU itself is under threat.

A new politics is needed: there are more activists now than ever before, though since activism these days involves sharing memes on Facebook and signing change.org petitions, the rise in political engagement may have been overstated. The ongoing battles over economic policy and defence of public services are, without doubt, important, but there are bigger battles to be fought.

Fascism again stalks the West, in both recognisable forms and new ones. In France, draconian restrictions on speech and assembly have followed the Paris shootings of November 2015; in Poland and Denmark, the far-right has gained unprecedented ground in elections. Meanwhile in America, Donald Trump clownishly suggests that as President, he might "go see Bill Gates [and talk to him about] closing that Internet up in some way. People will say 'Oh freedom of speech,' these are foolish people. We have a lot of foolish people."[101]

And sadly, Trump's comments closely match some from the British left who have chosen to shout FREEZEPEACH at people on social media who dare suggest that censorship might not be a good thing.

From left to right of the political spectrum, the task of

rebuilding liberalism is perhaps the most important one the West faces today. Free expression is not a fashionable thing to campaign for, but it needs to become one again. We must rediscover the Enlightenment.

References

Chapter 2

1. http://jewishchristianlit.com/Texts/ANEmrg/Inanna&
   Dumuzi.html
2. Pete Hamill, "Women on the Verge of a Legal Breakdown,"
   Playboy, January 1993, p189
3. http://www.climatechangenews.com/2015/04/14/twitter-
   failing-to-bridge-gap-between-climate-consensus-and-
   sceptics/

Chapter 3

4. Interview conducted with Polly Toynbee, a member of the
   Williams Committee

Chapter 4

5. Interview with Tuppy Owens, December 2011
6. Nadine Strossen, *Defending Pornography*, New York UP, 2000
   edition, p12
7. Nadine Strossen, *Defending Pornography*, p108
8. Andrea Dworkin, *Pornography: Men Possessing Women*,
   Plume, 1979, p23
9. Nadine Strossen, *Defending Pornography*, p23
10. David K. Johnson, *The Lavender Scare*, U of Chicago P, 2009,
    p58
11. Nadine Strossen, *Defending Pornography*, p110
12. Anthony D'Amato, "Porn Up, Rape Down," 2006
13. Edward de Grazia, *Girls Lean Back Everywhere: The Law of
    Obscenity and the Assault on Genius*, Vintage, 1992, p586
14. *The Voluntarist*, Vol. 3, No. 1, December 1984,
    http://voluntaryist.com/backissues/013.pdf
15. Nadine Strossen, *Defending Pornography*, p145
16. Brief of Feminists For Free Expression, amicus curiae,

Johnson v. County of Los Angeles Fire Department (filed in C.D. Cal. 1994), p16

17. Nadine Strossen, *Defending Pornography*, p206
18. Legs McNeil and Jennifer Osborne, *The Other Hollywood*, HarperCollins, 2005, p439
19. Catharine A. MacKinnon, *Toward a Feminist Theory of the State*, Harvard UP, 1989, p202
20. Catharine A. MacKinnon, *Only Words*, Harvard UP, 1993, p96
21. Gail Dines, *Pornland: How Porn Has Hijacked Our Sexuality*, Beacon Press, 2010, Chapter 3: From the Backstreet to Wall Street
22. http://www.forbes.com/2001/05/25/0524porn.html
23. http://internet-filter-review.toptenreviews.com/internet-pornography-statistics.html#anchor1
24. Gail Dines, *Pornland*, Chapter 2, p25
25. https://www.youtube.com/watch?v=PbJxTAYIxcU&feature=youtu.be
26. http://therealpornwikileaks.com/gail-dines-threatens-hotel-chain-with-blackmail/
27. Gail Dines, *Pornland*, p33
28. http://www.theguardian.com/commentisfree/2011/may/08/slutwalk-not-sexual-liberation

Chapter 5

29. In 2015, the Object website was taken offline without explanation
30. In 2015, the Object website was taken offline without explanation
31. http://www.drpetra.co.uk/blog/glamorous-careers-for-girls/
32. http://www.rightwingwatch.org/content/hagee-rock-music-satanic-cyanide-and-needs-be-taken-outside-and-burned
33. http://sexandcensorship.org/2014/10/letter-object-regarding-rape-allegations/
34. http://www.marieclaire.com/sex-love/a16474/women-porn-

habits-study/

35. http://www.christianitytoday.com/women/2013/july/why-i-tell-my-daughters-to-dress-modestly.html

36. Brooke Magnanti, *The Sex Myth: Why Everything We're Told Is Wrong*, W&N, 2012, Chapter 3

37. http://www.theguardian.com/society/2013/jun/17/sexualised-imagery-high-street

38. https://witness.theguardian.com/assignment/51bf3a24e4b04a1361c94e71

39. http://www.theguardian.com/culture/2013/jul/16/pornification-britains-high-streets

40. http://www.theguardian.com/uk/2006/nov/18/film.filmnews

41. Brooke Magnanti, *The Sex Myth*, Chapter 10

42. http://www.theguardian.com/lifeandstyle/2010/sep/10/kat-banyard-influential-young-feminist

Chapter 6

43. http://www.atvod.co.uk/uploads/files/For_Adults_Only_FINAL.pdf

44. http://sexandcensorship.org/2013/11/concerns-raised-child-protection-conference/

45. http://www.nytimes.com/2011/08/12/world/europe/12iht-social12.html?hpw&_r=0

46. http://www.theguardian.com/uk/2011/aug/08/london-riots-blackberry-messenger-looting

47. http://www.telegraph.co.uk/technology/news/8862335/Cameron-told-not-to-shut-down-internet.html

48. http://www.breitbart.com/london/2015/03/20/bbc-featured-block-bot-runs-into-legal-trouble/

49. http://www.bbc.com/news/uk-25641941

50. http://www.telegraph.co.uk/news/uknews/law-and-order/11627180/Five-internet-trolls-a-day-convicted-in-UK-as-figures-show-ten-fold-increase.html

51. http://www.bbc.co.uk/news/uk-29909981

52. http://blog.lemnsissay.com/2014/09/26/brett-baileys-exhibit-b-real-human-zoo/#sthash.dJgsNROe.dpbs

Chapter 7

53. http://www.losetheladsmags.org.uk/about/
54. http://moronwatch.net/2013/07/dear-co-op.html
55. https://en.wikipedia.org/wiki/Nuts_(magazine)
56. http://nomorepage3.org/faqss/
57. http://www.thatericalper.com/2013/02/10/on-grammy-night-lets-remember-how-far-weve-come-the-citizens-council-of-greater-new-orleans-flyer-from-1960s/
58. http://www.abc.net.au/news/2014-03-20/hamad-dont-call-beyonces-sexual-empowerment-feminism/5330918
59. http://www.theguardian.com/commentisfree/2013/aug/27/miley-cyrus-twerking-cultural-appropriation
60. http://www.theguardian.com/commentisfree/2013/nov/10/black-women-music-industry-sex
61. http://www.theguardian.com/commentisfree/2013/dec/13/sexed-up-music-videos-problem-beyonce
62. http://www.theguardian.com/culture/2013/nov/13/cliff-richard-miley-cyrus
63. http://www.theguardian.com/music/2014/jan/13/bbfc-wants-age-rating-system-introduced-online-videos
64. http://www.theguardian.com/commentisfree/2009/aug/30/pornography-corporate-responsibility-developing-world
65. http://www.un.org/africarenewal/magazine/january-2008/aids-deaths-are-declining-reports-un
66. http://asa.org.uk/About-ASA/About-regulation.aspx
67. http://asa.org.uk/Rulings/Adjudications/2013/7/Renault-UK-Ltd/SHP_ADJ_226910.aspx#.VTYUiBz3-iw
68. http://www.dailymail.co.uk/news/article-2366298/Renault-advert-banned-watchdog-treats-women-like-sexual-objects.html
69. https://www.change.org/p/no-to-sexist-ads

70. http://www.theguardian.com/lifeandstyle/2014/nov/19/julien-blanc-barred-entering-uk-pick-up-artist
71. http://www.theguardian.com/commentisfree/2014/nov/18/feminism-rosetta-scientist-shirt-dapper-laughs-julien-blanc-inequality
72. http://www.huffingtonpost.co.uk/2014/11/07/nigel-farage-russell-brand-parklife_n_6120012.html
73. http://www.worldmag.com/2015/03/actor_russell_brand_makes_anti_porn_appeal_but_google_isn_t_buying_it
74. http://www.managementtoday.co.uk/opinion/1340215/the-research-isnt-actually-research/
75. http://sexandcensorship.org/2013/11/sex-porn-addictive-david-ley/
76. http://www.huffingtonpost.com/2014/02/15/religious-people-addicted-to-porn_n_4794614.html
77. http://www.bbc.co.uk/news/education-32115162
78. https://www.facebook.com/conservatives/posts/10153019828284279
79. http://www.independent.co.uk/news/uk/the-government-is-trying-to-ban-anonymous-porn-viewing-10157943.html

Chapter 8

80. http://www.independent.co.uk/news/science/porn-stars-and-the-naked-truth-8348388.html
81. http://stakeholders.ofcom.org.uk/binaries/internet/explicit-material-vod.pdf
82. http://www.theguardian.com/society/2015/feb/24/teenage-pregnancy-england-wales-lowest-46-years
83. http://aic.gov.au/media_library/publications/proceedings/14/kutchinsky.pdf
84. https://www.washingtonpost.com/wp-dyn/content/article/2006/06/18/AR2006061800610.html
85. http://ojp.gov/newsroom/pressreleases/2013/ojppr030713.pdf

86. http://www.theglobeandmail.com/globe-debate/the-amazing-news-about-rape-statistics/article4200939/
87. Diamond M et al, "Pornography and sex crimes in the Czech Republic," *Archives of Sexual Behavior*, 2010, DOI 10.1007/s 10508-010-9696-y
88. http://www.slate.com/articles/sports/sports_nut/2011/08/unbreakable.html
89. gy-sexist-gender-stereotypes
90. http://sexandcensorship.org/2014/01/british-doomed-lonely/
91. http://idei.fr/sites/default/files/medias/doc/conf/sic/papers_2007/kendall.pdf

Chapter 9

92. https://www.rt.com/uk/170228-porn-filters-web-censorship/
93. http://www.wired.co.uk/news/archive/2015-01/20/sky-web-filtering
94. http://mancunion.com/2015/10/07/update-yiannopoulos-also-banned-from-censorship-event/
95. http://www.theguardian.com/housing-network/2013/nov/14/london-property-foreign-investors
96. http://www.theguardian.com/uk-news/davehillblog/2013/oct/27/london-population-changes-june-2012
97. http://geekfeminism.wikia.com/wiki/Safe_space
98. http://geekfeminism.wikia.com/wiki/Trigger_warning
99. http://www.unwomen.org/en/news/stories/2015/9/cyber-violence-report-press-release
100. http://www.demos.co.uk/press-release/demos-male-celebrities-receive-more-abuse-on-twitter-than-women-2/
101. http://globalnews.ca/news/2389914/donald-trump-thinks-he-can-call-bill-gates-and-have-him-close-the-internet/

Contemporary culture has eliminated both the concept of the public and the figure of the intellectual. Former public spaces – both physical and cultural – are now either derelict or colonized by advertising. A cretinous anti-intellectualism presides, cheerled by expensively educated hacks in the pay of multinational corporations who reassure their bored readers that there is no need to rouse themselves from their interpassive stupor. The informal censorship internalized and propagated by the cultural workers of late capitalism generates a banal conformity that the propaganda chiefs of Stalinism could only ever have dreamt of imposing. Zer0 Books knows that another kind of discourse – intellectual without being academic, popular without being populist – is not only possible: it is already flourishing, in the regions beyond the striplit malls of so-called mass media and the neurotically bureaucratic halls of the academy. Zer0 is committed to the idea of publishing as a making public of the intellectual. It is convinced that in the unthinking, blandly consensual culture in which we live, critical and engaged theoretical reflection is more important than ever before.

ZERO BOOKS

Capitalist Realism Is there no alternative?
Mark Fisher
An analysis of the ways in which capitalism has presented itself as
the only realistic political-economic system.
Paperback: November 27, 2009 978-1-84694-317-1 $14.95 £7.99.
eBook: July 1, 2012 978-1-78099-734-6 $9.99 £6.99.

The Wandering Who? A study of Jewish identity politics
Gilad Atzmon
An explosive unique crucial book tackling the issues of Jewish
Identity Politics and ideology and their global influence.
Paperback: September 30, 2011 978-1-84694-875-6 $14.95 £8.99.
eBook: September 30, 2011 978-1-84694-876-3 $9.99 £6.99.

Clampdown Pop-cultural wars on class and gender
Rhian E. Jones
Class and gender in Britpop and after, and why 'chav' is a
feminist issue.
Paperback: March 29, 2013 978-1-78099-708-7 $14.95 £9.99.
eBook: March 29, 2013 978-1-78099-707-0 $7.99 £4.99.

The Quadruple Object
Graham Harman
Uses a pack of playing cards to present Harman's metaphysical
system of fourfold objects, including human access, Heidegger's
indirect causation, panpsychism and ontography.
Paperback: July 29, 2011 978-1-84694-700-1 $16.95 £9.99.

Weird Realism Lovecraft and Philosophy
Graham Harman
As Hölderlin was to Martin Heidegger and Mallarmé to Jacques
Derrida, so is H.P. Lovecraft to the Speculative Realist philoso-
phers.
Paperback: September 28, 2012 978-1-78099-252-5 $24.95 £14.99.
eBook: September 28, 2012 978-1-78099-907-4 $9.99 £6.99.

Sweetening the Pill or How We Got Hooked on Hormonal Birth
Control
Holly Grigg-Spall
Is it really true? Has contraception liberated or oppressed
women?
Paperback: September 27, 2013 978-1-78099-607-3 $22.95 £12.99.
eBook: September 27, 2013 978-1-78099-608-0 $9.99 £6.99.

Why Are We The Good Guys? Reclaiming Your Mind From The
Delusions Of Propaganda
David Cromwell
A provocative challenge to the standard ideology that Western
power is a benevolent force in the world.
Paperback: September 28, 2012 978-1-78099-365-2 $26.95 £15.99.
eBook: September 28, 2012 978-1-78099-366-9 $9.99 £6.99.

The Truth about Art Reclaiming quality
Patrick Doorly
The book traces the multiple meanings of art to their various
sources, and equips the reader to choose between them.
Paperback: August 30, 2013 978-1-78099-841-1 $32.95 £19.99.

Bells and Whistles More Speculative Realism
Graham Harman
In this diverse collection of sixteen essays, lectures, and inter-
views Graham Harman lucidly explains the principles of

Speculative Realism, including his own object-oriented philosophy.
Paperback: November 29, 2013 978-1-78279-038-9 $26.95 £15.99.
eBook: November 29, 2013 978-1-78279-037-2 $9.99 £6.99.

Towards Speculative Realism: Essays and Lectures Essays and Lectures
Graham Harman
These writings chart Harman's rise from Chicago sportswriter to co founder of one of Europe's most promising philosophical movements: Speculative Realism.
Paperback: November 26, 2010 978-1-84694-394-2 $16.95 £9.99.
eBook: January 1, 1970 978-1-84694-603-5 $9.99 £6.99.

Meat Market Female flesh under capitalism
Laurie Penny
A feminist dissection of women's bodies as the fleshy fulcrum of capitalist cannibalism, whereby women are both consumers and consumed.
Paperback: April 29, 2011 978-1-84694-521-2 $12.95 £6.99.
eBook: May 21, 2012 978-1-84694-782-7 $9.99 £6.99.

Translating Anarchy The Anarchism of Occupy Wall Street
Mark Bray
An insider's account of the anarchists who ignited Occupy Wall Street.
Paperback: September 27, 2013 978-1-78279-126-3 $26.95 £15.99.
eBook: September 27, 2013 978-1-78279-125-6 $6.99 £4.99.

One Dimensional Woman
Nina Power
Exposes the dark heart of contemporary cultural life by examining pornography, consumer capitalism and the ideology of women's work.

Paperback: November 27, 2009 978-1-84694-241-9 $14.95 £7.99.
eBook: July 1, 2012 978-1-78099-737-7 $9.99 £6.99.

Dead Man Working
Carl Cederstrom, Peter Fleming
An analysis of the dead man working and the way in which
capital is now colonizing life itself.
Paperback: May 25, 2012 978-1-78099-156-6 $14.95 £9.99.
eBook: June 27, 2012 978-1-78099-157-3 $9.99 £6.99.

Unpatriotic History of the Second World War
James Heartfield
The Second World War was not the Good War of legend. James
Heartfield explains that both Allies and Axis powers fought for
the same goals - territory, markets and natural resources.
Paperback: September 28, 2012 978-1-78099-378-2 $42.95 £23.99.
eBook: September 28, 2012 978-1-78099-379-9 $9.99 £6.99.

Find more titles at www.zero-books.net